T0077956

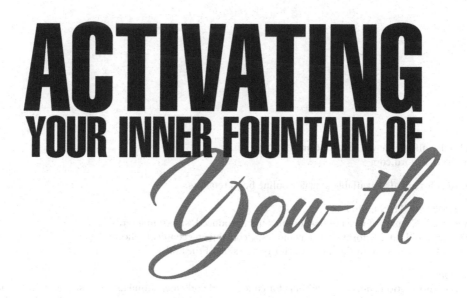

ACTIVATING
YOUR INNER FOUNTAIN OF
You-th

New Discoveries In
Anti-Aging & Longevity

Joy Peters, PhD

Order this book online at www.trafford.com
or email orders@trafford.com

Most Trafford titles are also available at major online book retailers.

Print information available on the last page.

ISBN: 978-1-6987-0407-4 (sc)
ISBN: 978-1-6987-0406-7 (e)

Trafford rev. 12/19/2020

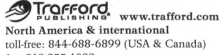

North America & international
toll-free: 844-688-6899 (USA & Canada)
fax: 812 355 4082

Table of Contents

Chapter 1

The Search For The Fountain Of Youth

The Fountain of Youth

Since the dawn of time, people have long sought to find the mysterious fountain of youth. From the days of Cleopatra to Ponce De Leon, both searched till their deaths for this infamous fountain of youth and the search has continued, thereafter.

Basically, the reason why the search continues for the fountain of youth is because legend has it that if one drinks from this magical spring immortality is within its waters, the fountain of youth is a magic anti-aging elixir that if you skinny-dip in it, the bathier may submerge as an old person an transform beneath these magical waters so when they emerge, they walk away forever young. For centuries, legend has told that drinking from the fountain of youth, restored the body back to its most attractive and youthful state.

Early explorers of the fountain of youth, described in artist renderings depictions of older adults walking into this magical fountain of youth and exiting out on the other side of the banks of this pool of water, as young and energetic as a vibrant teen. Were these early photos real or mythological? The depictions sent many explorers on expeditions around the globe in search of this magical or mythical pond. Some say anti-aging waters do exist. In reality, these youth baths were likely pools of water, such as naturally occurring hot-springs or cold glacial mountain run off that contain minerals or naturally occurring substances such as marine algae or other compounds that help stimulate cell and DNA repair. Could the explorers discover cool spring water wells, underground springs or glacial water artisans that are all pristine water sources that are abundantly rich in life giving minerals.

Anti-Aging Peat Moors

In several areas of Europe, there are peat moor bogs that are said to have incredibly powerful anti-aging properties. Within these moss swamp-like wetlands, human corpses have been found with beautifully preserved skin that made investigators believe the corpses were only recently deceased but when the forensic lab report returned to the police, it was revealed, by carbon-dating that the body was actually thousands of years old! How can a 2000 yr old body be preserved in a way that the skin is so beautiful and completely intact and so fresh as to fool seasoned murder investigators into thinking the body has only just recently been deceased for maybe only a couple of weeks? Scientists determined that the secret was in the bog itself, the types of plants and the organic acids, with its naturally occurring pH level similar to vinegar, preserving the human bodies in the same way as preserving foods by pickling as sort of a natural embalming fluid. It is believed there are fountain of youth properties located in the organic compounds of the mud in these bogs that have yet to be harnessed as a fountain of youth for the living.

Elixir Of Life A Magic Drink

The elixir of life, also known as the elixir of immortality and sometimes equated to the philosopher's stone. Legend has it that it is a potion that grants the drinker eternal life and/or eternal youth. This elixir was also said to cure all diseases. Alchemists in various ages and cultures sought to formulate the elixir. The concept originated in ancient India or China where the concept preceded that in Europe for many millennia.

Cleopatra's Secret "Giver of Life" The Nile

Legend has it that Cleopatra's most esteemed beauty was sourced from the river Nile. She lived beside the Nile and basked in its lush untainted waters like a fountain of youth. It is said that she frequently enjoyed many baths sourced from the mineral rich Nile and it's qualities are famed to be a fountain of youth and was dubbed by the Egyptian people and gods as the "Giver Of Life".

The Source Of Your Inner Fountain Of Youth

Up to 70% of the human adult body is water. The brain and heart are composed of 73% water, and the lungs are about 83% water. The skin contains 64% water, the muscles and kidneys are 79% water, and even the bones are watery with the marrow being 31% water. Therefore, it is logical to say our body itself is an internal fountain of youth.

Your Inner Fountain Of Youth

Today, scientists have made real anti-aging discoveries, and now, you don't need to find a magic pond or potion to have youthful vitality, good health and longevity as the fountain of youth lies within you, in fact a fountain of youth is hidden in the DNA coding of each and every one of us. Science has proven that not only does beauty come from within, but the genes for longevity are hidden within us and it is possible to resurrect the mechanisms of youthful vitality from within if we do the right things. According to researchers our DNA can be tweaked for longer life extension which may help your body keep its youthful vigor and vitality for an extended lifetime.

Today's Modern Search For Eternal Beauty

In the search for everlasting youth, many seek to buy their everlasting beauty in a jar. Yet despite the personal care products industry pouring multi-billion dollars yearly into the development of new products, most pre-2020 skin creams and serums on the market simply do not deliver the age-defying results they promise. There has been little hope until the most recent discoveries in aging research which prove aging is from a failure of internal processes that eventually lose youthful function within. However, most recently, longevity researchers have discovered new ways to reactivate the processes, internally and to stimulate the external skin to repair itself as youthful skin does, too. This can best be done internally, vrs externally according to the age scientists and they say that it may be possible to reverse our skin's timeline at the cellular level since the discovery of hidden culprits that act as "cellular boogie-men compounds" such as, bad proteins that cause wrinkles and have discovered new compounds that halt the age-related damage and slow the ever shortening of our age-clock, the DNA strand telomeres. The most advanced age scientists have also discovered ways to neutralize the causes of the ravages of time and how to lengthen human telomeres thus extending the length of the human lifespan and immortal beauty. Allowing these nerdy scientists to become the coolest people on the planet. You can find out who these scientists are by doing a search of the top ivy league age research laboratories worldwide or looking through the NIH research files but within these pages you will discover the basics of how to feel and look younger with these cutting-edge anti-aging discoveries that the celebrities do plus additional natural anti-aging home tips that help stimulate the fountain of youth within your very own body.

Beauty Begins On The Inside And Is An Outward Reflection Of Your Inner Health

The Secret To Activating Your Inner Fountain Of Youth

The most important thing to activate your inner fountain of youth and to age more youthfully is by following a sensible daily age reversing protocol that will help you better control the way you age. These basics can not only prevent and reverse chronic illnesses but also the signs and symptoms of aging.

Key Tips To Activate Your Inner Fountain Of Youth

Activating your inner fountain of youth doesn't have to be an overwhelming task. It can be as simple as changing the things you do to yourself because the damage that we do to ourselves with bad habits, are the easiest things to correct. There are a number of ways that you can activate your body's self-healing mechanisms and optimize your health while prolonging the time left on your biological clock to extend your life-span.

- **Step One** The first step of the reverse aging program deals with making dietary changes, boosting the immune system, reducing systemic inflammation and removing toxic waste from the body- all pretty basic stuff. In other words, this part of the damage control is up to you. You are in charge and play an active role in how effectively you can reverse aging, but more about that in later chapters.
- **Step Two** The second part of damage control involves preventing and reversing damage at the cellular level. This component of reverse aging may not totally be up to you as factors promoting aging are genetically programmed in your cells. Having said that, there are still some proactive measures you can take to prevent damage at the cellular level.

  - you can incorporate more exercise into your daily routine to keep circulation moving, the heart pumping well, and the lymphatic system flowing freely. This will, among other things, nourish and replenish your cells well.
  - you can invest in some quality anti-aging products that will work internally to regenerate cells and minimize aging effects. A lot more on this in upcoming chapters.

- **Step Three** The final step in this process addresses hormonal changes that affect aging at a macro level. Hormones are the body's chemical messengers telling the body what to do and when. With regards to aging, hormones tell the body how to age and any fluctuations in hormonal levels affects aging.

- ○ While hormonal production cannot be completely dominated by any single treatment, you can make small but sensible changes to restore these imbalances. Some basics to boost the body's ability to create and balance hormones include changing lifestyle and dietary habits while staying away from common stressors and detoxifying.
- ○ Consider hormonal therapy.

Longevity And The Inner Fountain Of Youth

Longevity is having a long lifespan. Longevity is those who live longer than an average lifespan. Life expectancy has increased significantly worldwide but the new goal is with a longer life expectancy to stay healthy and as youthful as possible throughout our entire lives so we have a better quality of life. It is an important goal for those who strive for Longevity that during their end of life phase they seek to avoid the need for drugs and surgeries while reducing the risk of becoming infantile or bed ridden or unable to care for ourselves in the end. It is possible there are many who seem to escape the ravages of time and look 20 years younger than they really are. Some would say the long liver's have good genes or that they follow a strict diet and healthy living practices but in interviewing some of these long-liver's it becomes obvious that they aren't always doing all the right things. Some of them smoke, some of them eat fried foods, some occasionally drink alcohol, still they live long lives. There is something special within their bodies that is the secret to longevity and it is the key to activating a flowing inner fountain of youth, too.

Your Blood Is A River Of Life And Part Of Your Inner Fountain Of Youth.

Your Blood

You have eight pints of blood flowing through your veins like a river and without this raging river of life, we cannot live. Your blood is part of your inner fountain of youth, it delivers oxygen and nutrients to all of your cells, organs and tissues to keep us alive and deliver all of the components necessary for the body to continue to repair and regenerate itself. Your blood consists of liquids and solids compounds that are the essential building blocks of life.

- The liquid part of your blood is called plasma, it is made of water, salts and protein. Over half of your blood is plasma.

- The solid part of your blood contains red blood cells, white blood cells and platelets.

Blood contains:

- **Plasma**- cells make antibodies to fight bacteria and viruses, to stop infection and disease constitutes 55% of total blood volume.
- **White Blood Cells**- There are 8,000 white cells per cubic millimetre of blood, they are made in your bone marrow and are part of your immune system and they help your body fight off infections and other diseases.
- **Platelets**- or thrombocytes form in your bone marrow and play a major role in blood clotting that helps prevent bleeding to death during a serious wound.
- **Red Blood Cells**- have over 20,000 receptor sites, the majority deliver oxygen and nutrients to the body the other 2,000 pick up and carry metabolic waste to the liver and kidneys to be eliminated thus aiding in detoxification.

Your Blood's Role In Life Expectancy

Females have a life-span expectancy of living up to five years longer than males on average. There are several reasons why but one of the main reasons is from the accumulation of Iron-Oxide3 in the blood. Iron-Oxide3 is a rust-like toxic form of iron that can bind with cholesterol and form plaque in the arteries and then lead to strokes later on in life. It is believed that a males shorter life-expectancy is because they tend to have an increased level and a greater buildup of iron-oxide 3 in the blood that it leads to a higher risk of strokes while women eliminate iron-oxide through menstruation throughout their adult lives which men have no additional biological means of eliminating it. However, after menopause women also begin to build up iron oxide at the same rate as women. The good news is you can help the body eliminate by doing a heavy metal detox cleanse at least once a year. You should also take a seasonal heavy metal detox bath at least four times each year. That being said, Iron is necessary for healthy blood, but there is a good type of iron and a bad type of iron.

Hemoglobin The Self-Healing Blood Component

In addition to transporting oxygen, hemoglobin carries carbon dioxide out of the cells and into the lungs. Carbon dioxide is then exhaled as a person breathes. Having low hemoglobin can make it difficult for the body to perform these functions.

Symptoms of low hemoglobin levels include:

- Fatigue
- Easy bruising
- Shortness of breath
- Irregular heartbeat
- Pale skin and gums
- Muscle weakness
- Recurring headaches

Benefits Of Increasing Hemoglobin

Hemoglobin also contributes to homeostasis in the body and its ability to maintain a healthy biochemical balance. The blood's buffering capacity, ATP (the spark of life enzyme) and NO (nitric oxide) are released from red blood cells and contributes to vasodilation and improved blood flow to working muscles. These functions require adequate amounts of red blood cells in circulation. You can improve levels of hemoglobin by eating more iron-rich foods. Iron works to boost the production of hemoglobin, which also helps to form more red blood cells. Also do the following to increase your hemoglobin levels:

- Huggs
- Exercise
- Therapeutic massage
- Eat iron-rich foods

Your Blood Type

Knowing your blood type is one more way to better understand and manage your health. Your blood type is usually the same as one of your parents, it is a genetic gift that cannot be altered. It is crucial to know and to make healthy choices to support your blood type. Eating foods that are more compatible to the enzymes in your blood type may be more digestible and better absorbed. By eating a diet that is in accordance to your specific type your diet can have a better impact on maintaining your good health and keeping your blood healthy. Considering your blood type to make dietary decisions according to your blood type may help reduce various disease risks related to your individual health.

Blood Type And Longevity

Your blood type can alter your reaction to food substances and in some, eating the wrong foods may create various reactions and special sensitivities to various food substances. It is worth reading about special recommendations for your specific blood type. A blood endotype test can quickly reveal your blood type. There are eight main blood types:

- A+
- A-
- B+
- B-
- O+
- O-
- AB+
- AB-

Knowing your blood type can be crucial in a medical emergency, but it can also offer some interesting insight into your health. See how your blood type might play a role in your well-being, based on results of some recent studies.

Best Longevity Foods For Your Type A-O Blood Types:

- **A+ & A-**

    o fruit, vegetables, tofu, seafood, turkey, and whole grains but avoid meat.
    o weight-loss foods: seafood, vegetables, pineapple, olive oil, and soy.
    o Avoid dairy, wheat, corn, and kidney beans.

- **B+ & B-**

    o meat, fruit, dairy, seafood, and grains.
    o Weight-loss foods- green vegetables, eggs and daily licorice tea.
    o Avoid chicken, corn, peanuts, and wheat.

- **O+ & O-**

    o high-protein foods, meat, vegetables, fish, and fruit but limit grains, beans, and legumes.
    o Weight-loss, seafood, kelp, red meat, broccoli, spinach, and olive oil are best;
    o Avoid wheat, corn, and dairy

- **AB+ & AB-**

  - Eat dairy, tofu, lamb, fish, grains, fruit, and vegetables.
  - For AB- weight loss: tofu, seafood, green vegetables, and kelp are best but chicken, corn, buckwheat, and kidney beans should be avoided.

Specifics About Your Blood Type

- **A+** your blood contains type A antigens with the protein rhesus (Rh) factor.
- **A-** platelets are called the 'universal platelet type' and you do not have the Rh protein.
- **B+** there is very high demand for your B+ blood. People with sickle cell anemia and thalassemia need regular transfusions. Consider donations if you are B+ subtype Ro.
- **B-** you can only receive blood from other B- donors or from type O- donors. Only 2% of the population have B- B blood types originated some 3.5 million years ago, from a genetic mutation that modified one of the sugars that sit on the surface of red blood cells therefore all B blood types should take measures to avoid inflammation.
- **O+** You have the most common blood type. 38% of the population has O+ blood
- **O-** You are a universal blood donor. O-negative: African-American: 4 percent. Asian: 1 percent. Caucasian: 8 percent.
- **AB+** You have both A and B antigens at the surface of your red blood cells so you are a universal plasma donor. AB blood group is the result of the intermingling between Caucasian (commonly group A) and Mongolian (commonly group B) people
- **AB-** You have the newest and rarest blood type. Less than 1% of the U.S. population have AB negative blood, making it the least common blood type among Americans. Finding donors can be a challenge. AB-negative: African-American: 0.3 percent. Asian: 0.1 percent. Caucasian: 1 percent.

Rare Blood Type Discovery

Another rare blood type has emerged and is most common in the ethnic groups: African American: U-negative and Duffy-negative blood types. Native American and Alaskan native: RzRz, also known as Rh-null or the "golden blood" type.

Blood Type And Risk For Disease

Your blood type is just one factor that contributes to your risk for certain health conditions. "While your blood type may put you at a higher risk for certain conditions, nothing is definitive. Being aware of how your blood type may impact your health is a good start, but it's also important to see your physician for regular check-ups and maintain a healthy lifestyle. Your blood type may put you at a higher risk for some medical conditions, as follows:

- **Blood Type And Heart Disease**
  People with type O have the lowest risk for heart disease but everyone should still take measures to protect their heart health. People with AB and B blood types are at the greatest risk of heart disease, which could be a result of higher rates of inflammation. A heart-healthy diet and lifestyle is very important for people with AB and B blood types.

- **Blood Type And Cancer**
  A healthy lifestyle that focuses on preventing inflammation and eating a cancer-fighting diet is paramount to longevity and good health, which can also help reduce your risk for developing cancer. Studies have found that people with blood type A or AB are at higher risk for stomach cancer while people with A, B or AB blood types may have an increased risk for pancreatic cancer.

- **Blood Type And Stress**
  Everyone should take steps to reduce anxiety and stress and have a low stress lifestyle to stay healthy. Especially, those with type A as studies show A types tend to have heightened levels of cortisol and elevated stress hormones in the body. There is more to the meaning of an A type personality, literally if the person is also an A blood type. If you have type A blood, with high-stress and have trouble handling stress, it is imperative for you to take stress lowering measures in daily life to lower their risk of future stress related health problems. However, stress management is important for all blood types.

Having "Good Blood" And Longevity

It is important to keep a check on your blood health. Regular labs are important for early detection of blood imbalances. Some clinics offer live blood assessment and often these types of tests can detect imbalances before a lab profile can. Additionally, various imbalances can be seen in live blood cell analysis prior to the development of an associated disease.

Cleaning Dirty Blood

Inflammation and Fibrin are two prime causes of aging and disease. It creates stagnation and sluggishness in the blood and throughout the body. Fibrin decreases the body's flexibility and inflammation accumulates and dulls youthful appearance. Fibrin is a tough protein arranged in long fibrous chains. It is formed from fibrinogen, a soluble protein that is produced by the liver that is found in blood plasma. Fibrin tends to form blockages that create barriers against the absorption of healing nutrients around areas of inflammation. Systemic enzymes can help clean up dirty blood.

Normal Blood Pressure Blood

The body's normal adult blood pressure (BP) is 120/80 mm these are considered normal blood pressure numbers. Blood pressure numbers above 129 systolic and over 80 diastolic are considered elevated. High BP can damage your veins and arteries which is the transport system of your blood, AKA river of life and fountain of youth this is why maintaining a healthy blood pressure is essential to anti-aging.

Good Blood Oxygen Level

Your blood oxygen levels are important to your health and are a major component in activating your inner fountain of youth, a pulse oximeter is used to measure your blood oxygen level. A normal reading is a Sp02 level that's between 95 and 100 percent oxygen. Cells die when oxygen levels are low. Low oxygen symptoms include:

- Yawning
- Fatigue
- Sluggish
- Tired
- Sleepy
- Blue coloring
- Cold hands and feet

To increase your levels of oxygen:

- Exercise
- Supplemental oxygen
- Drink more water H2O
- Hyperbaric Chamber Therapy

Your Blood Type And Genes

Your blood type is related to your heart, since your heart pumps blood to the rest of your body and blood type can put some people at a higher risk for conditions such as heart attack and heart disease. This is because of the ABO gene. The ABO gene is present in people with A, B, or AB blood types. The only blood type that doesn't have the ABO gene is type O. Read chapter five for more information about your genes. Your blood type is just one factor that contributes to your risk for certain health conditions. "While your blood type may put you at a higher risk for certain conditions, nothing is definitive. Being aware of how your blood type may impact your health is a good start, but it's also just as important to see your physician for regular check-ups and maintain a healthy lifestyle. Although the ABO gene may add a higher risk of cancer, and it can sometimes be hard to know which types of cancer. However, people with Type A blood have been found to have a higher risk of stomach cancer specifically, compared to those with other blood types but there are many effective preventative solutions to help decrease your genetic risk factors but your inner fountain of youth is not only related to your blood, there's more to your inner fountain of youth than just your blood. The centenarians, those who live over 100 years have their secrets but the super centenarians have even more longevity secrets to share, those are the souls who live to be a ripe old age of 105+ years.

Blood & Genetic Test Results Of The Oldest Documented Woman

An analysis of the blood samples of the oldest documented woman, Jeanne Calment, indicated that her blood levels were in the normal ranges up until she was 114 years old. At that age, she showed no signs of dehydration, anemia, chronic infection or renal impairment. Genetic analysis of her HLA system revealed the presence of the DR1 Allele. HLA-DR1 (DR1) is a serotype that recognizes the DRB1 gene products. It has been observed to be common in centenarians, people who live over 100 years of age.

"Healthy Blood Is Important, But The Real Quest In Anti-Aging Is Learning How To Activate Your Inner Fountain of Youth".

Secrets Of A Super-Centenarian

A Supercentenarian is someone who has reached the age of 110. This age is achieved by about one in a thousand centenarians. Centenarians are those who live to be over 100 years old. Supercentenarians tend to live ten years longer than centenarians and also live a life typically free of major age-related diseases. Over 1,500 super-centenarians have been documented in history. Many others have claimed to have lived to age 110 and with today's advancements in genetic medicine it is possible to live well beyond centenarian status.

Living Beyond Super-Centenarian Is A Super-Human Super-Power

Longest Living Supercentenarian Humans

The oldest person ever documented was Jeanne Calment (1875–1997) of France, who lived to the age of 122 years old. Her age was independently verified and the oldest man ever recorded was Jiroemon Kimura who lived to 116 years old in Japan.

- Oldest Female-Age 122- Jeanne Calment - France
- Oldest Male-Age 116- Jiroemon Kimura- Japan

We will explore the life and lifestyles of these two, the longest living man and longest living woman. We will review their culture, their lifestyle, the environment they lived in and personal habits.

Vive La France! Joie De Vivre!

The French saying Joie Devivre, means "the joy of life" and maybe they have found a longevity secret in this philosophy of life. Vive La France is another common saying which means "long live France". Put them together and you will quickly see a culture whose ultimate aim is to have a happy long life! The French do have a special appreciation for the enjoyment of life that is to be admired and we could all benefit from many of their habits, such as small portion size, not too much salt or sugar and the use of bitters which satisfies the palette, quelches the appetite for food and help in weight control. The French also have appreciation for the arts, music, theater, a propensity to have fun in song and dance and other forms of entertainment. The women have natural beauty and confidence. They love to stimulate their senses with the finest perfumes and wines. The French have made many scientific discoveries and contributions to the advancement of mankind, including research in anti-aging and the discovery of microbes and the pasteurization of bacteria.

Life Details Of Oldest Living Woman

- **Jeanne Calmet - Age 122**

  - She was from France
  - She lived with her parents from birth till marriage
  - She lived in the Rhone river region of France.
  - She enjoyed painting, and playing piano.
  - She had hobbies such as fencing, cycling, tennis, swimming and rollerskating.
  - Jeanne Calment reportedly ascribed her longevity and youthful appearance to a diet rich in olive oil.
  - All her life she took care of her skin with olive oil and a puff of white rice powder.
  - She married at 21, and her husband's wealth allowed her to live without ever working.
  - She had a child, a daughter. Later was a grandmother who raised her grandson after her daughter died from pleurisy at age 36.
  - She and her husband would vacation at Uriage, France, mountaineering and enjoy the thermal waters there that contain sulphide and salt and have a molecular concentration similar to that of human blood serum which is unique in the world.
  - At Uriage spa, there are various curing techniques including showers, baths, hydromassages, applications of mud, filiform shower and aerosols.
  - She rode a bike and cycled for many years.
  - Later in life, Calment outlived all her family.
  - Her husband died at age 73 of cherry poisoning.
  - She entered an assisted care home at 112 and followed a scheduled daily ritual.
  - She woke at 6:45 am, and started the day with a long prayer at her window, thanking God for being alive and for the beautiful day which was starting.
  - She did gymnastics wearing her stereo headset. Her exercises included flexing and extending the hands then the legs.

- ○ Nurses noted that she moved faster than other residents who were 30 years younger.
- ○ Her breakfast consisted of coffee with milk and rusk.
- ○ She washed herself with a flannel cloth using soap and then applying olive oil to her face and body and then applying powder to her face.
- ○ She enjoyed braised beef daube
- ○ She didn't care for broiled fish.
- ○ She had dessert with every meal
- ○ She said that given a choice she would eat fried and spicy foods instead of bland foods.
- ○ She made herself fruit salads with bananas and oranges, daily.
- ○ She enjoyed dark chocolate, sometimes eating two pounds of dark chocolate per week.
- ○ After an evening meal on occasion, she drank a small glass of port wine
- ○ In the afternoon she would listen to the news on the radio, nap and then visit her neighbors telling them about news.
- ○ At nightfall she would dine, listen to music, enjoy a crossword puzzle.
- ○ Go to bed at 10:00 pm
- ○ She went to church weekly
- ○ She regularly conversed with God.
- ○ She spoke of and wondered about the afterlife.
- ○ Her tranquil state of mind probably contributed to her long life she said when she turned 112, "That's why they call me Calm-ent"
- ○ Jeanne was known for her wit, and felt that her sense of humour also played its part in her remarkable longevity.
- ○ At her 120th birthday, journalists asked her what kind of future she expected and she replied. "A very short one".
- ○ She remained clear thinking up to the day she passed away in 1997 at age 122 years.
- ○ Some skeptics tried to say she wasnt that old but her age was verified by 3 major research organizations confirming her status as the oldest documented woman to have lived, thus far.

Daily Fountain Of Youth Wake Up Drink

Upon waking each morning after overnight fasting, drink this drink to cleanse your palate and prep your digestive track for the day for autophagy and detoxification.

- • 1 Quart Boiling Water
- • 1 T. Turmeric Tea

- 1 T. Cinnamon
- 1 T. Chinese 5 Spice
- 1 T. Organic Earl Grey Tea
- 1 T. Optional Organic Coffee

Pour boiling water into a french-press, add tea or coffee, add spices, Stir. Press, Pour, Enjoy! It is also important to drink 32 ounces of plain water or a cup of warm lemon water each morning, too.

Mornings are for drinking!

Chapter 2
Your Inner Age Clock

Your Age Clock

Your age clock is regulated by your body's circadian rhythm, a natural, internal process that regulates the sleep-wake cycle and organ repair cycles which repeat on a nightly basis with each rotation of the Earth, roughly every 24 hours. Thus, when speaking of the circadian rhythm, it can refer to any biological process that displays an endogenous, entrainable oscillation of the earth's rotation, about 24 hours.

It is important to know that your body only goes through cell renewal and regeneration in the deeper states of sleep and every organ system takes a turn in repairing itself at different times during this cycle, as well. During an organ systems repair and regeneration time, the body shifts its energy into focusing on repairing one system at a time, once complete the repair mechanisms shift focus to another one until all systems are maintenced. Sleep disruptions interrupt the repair cycles and eventually lead to dysfunction and disease. Allowing the circadian rhythms to run their schedule uninterrupted is very important to your good health.

Night Time Is The Right Time To Repair Time

The circadian clock plays a role in your body's physical repair, mental processes, and behavior. It is part of your biological clock that regulates wake sleep cycles of bodily functions, it also responds to light and dark. There are four biological rhythms:

- circadian rhythms: a 24-hour cycle of physiological and behavioral rhythms, such as, sleeping.
- infradian rhythms: are biological rhythms that last longer than 24 hours, such as metabolism
- diurnal rhythms: the circadian rhythm synced with day and night a repeating sinusoidal curve opposite of nocturnal.

- ultradian rhythms: biological rhythms with a shorter period and higher frequency than circadian rhythms such as, such as a menstrual cycle and ovulation.

Your mind and body need sleep to stay healthy. Your body is made to sleep at night. This is why we don't have adaptations like night vision and an enhanced sense of smell and hearing like nocturnal animals do. The brain and body become exhausted when we tamper with our circadian rhythms for example more auto accidents occur before daylight. This is the reason we need 8 hours of sleep each night to maintain optimal mind-body functions.

Age Clock Regulators

In order to turn back the hands of time on your age clock and sustain a lifelong inner fountain of youth there are three body systems you must strive to keep in balance.

1. Circadian Rhythms
2. Chemistry Balance
3. Hormone Balance

If you keep these three systems in balance, your body stays in a state of homeostasis and will properly regulate all other systems in the body, such as the blood vascular system, digestive system and immune system. The two systems that you must strive to keep in balance is your:

1. Endocrine system - Regulates hormone balance
2. Metabolic system - Regulates metabolic balance

Hormonal Endocrine System

Hormones are involved in every aspect of your health. Your body needs very specific amounts or each hormone for your organs to maintain good health and proper function. Your endocrine system is the hormone system, it is composed of organs and glands that produce and regulate hormones within the body. For example, insulin is a hormone produced by your pancreas, an endocrine organ that regulates your blood sugar levels. The endocrine system has many glands and organs that release a steady stream of hormones and maintain hormonal balance unless something triggers an imbalance. The endocrine system is a compensatory system so these glands can compensate for each other. The organs and glands of the Endocrine system are:

- Thyroid- Metabolism
- Parathyroid- Calcium uptake/chemistry balance
- Hypothalamus- Molecules of emotion
- Stomach- Digestion
- Duodenum- Absorption of nutrients
- Jejunum- Absorbs amino acids, and fatty acids
- Pancreas- Absorbs & regulates blood sugar levels
- Pineal Gland-regulates melatonin in light-dark cycles
- Pituitary Gland - the 'master gland' as the hormones it produces control the thyroid, adrenals, ovaries, and testes.
- Thymus- T cells and Immunity
- Testes (in men) - Reproduction/Sperm
- Ovaries (in women) - Reproduction/Eggs
- Kidneys- Eliminate liquid toxins, maintain homeostasis balance chemistry.
- Adrenal Glands- Stress hormones and survival.

Hormonal imbalances may increase your risk of:

- Obesity,
- Diabetes,
- Heart disease and
- Other health problems.

In the past, aging and other age related factors were often beyond our control until now, and the good news is, recent scientific discoveries have found that there are many steps you can take to turn back the hands of time, look years younger and to help maintain your hormonal balance and function as you age, gracefully and feel younger, forever. The following can help improve your hormonal health:

- Consuming nutritious foods
- Exercising on a regular daily basis
- Engaging in healthy lifestyle behaviors

Biological Rhythm Imbalances & Disorders

Biological rhythm imbalances lead to various health disorders that can affect a person's sense of well-being and health. Some of the negative effects of an imbalance include:

- Anxiety

- Loss of Mental clarity
- Fatigue
- Daytime tiredness
- Seasonal affective disorder
- Depression
- Lowered stamina and performance
- Accident-prone
- Increased risk of diabetes
- Weight gain and obesity

Adrenal Burnout

Adrenal fatigue is not technically an accepted medical diagnosis. It is a lay term applied to a collection of nonspecific symptoms, such as body aches, fatigue, nervousness.

High Cortisol- Longevity Enemy # 1

Cortisol is the Dr. Jeckle/Mr. Hyde hormone. Most bodily cells have cortisol receptors and cortisol has a controlling effect on salt and water balance in the body. However, this good guy/bad guy hormone affects a vast variety of other functions in the body.

Cortisol can help:

- Control blood sugar levels,
- Regulate metabolism,
- Help reduce inflammation, and
- Assist with memory formulation
- Helps regulate blood pressure
- Helps you react during emergency

Too much cortisol can cause:

- Adrenal burn out & Exhaustion
- Rapid weight gain
- Fat accumulation face, chest and abdomen
- A red flushed face.
- High blood pressure
- Blotchy skin changes

- Easy to bruise
- Purple stretch marks
- Muscle weakness
- Mood swings
- Anxiety
- Depression
- Irritability
- Cushing syndrome
- A fatty hump between your shoulders,
- A rounded face, and
- Stretch marks on your skin
- High blood pressure
- Bone loss
- Type 2 diabetes.

Lifestyle Tips To Lower High Cortisol

Some simple lifestyle tips to help lower high cortisol levels and have more energy and improved health are:

- Get Adequate Sleep
- Exercise, but don't over-exercise
- Quelch Stressful Thinking
- Recognize Anxiety & Learn to Relax
- Maintain Healthy Relationships
- Have More Fun.
- Do more things that you enjoy doing
- Drink water
- Eat a healthy diet
- Change situations that upset you
- Make some healthy changes

Eat A Cortisol Lowering Diet

Avoid all foods that increase your cortisol levels.

The following foods spike cortisol:

- Vegetable and Seed Oil (hexene toxins)
- Hexene triggers inflammation and cortisol

- ○ Flavored Yogurt
- ○ Trans-Fats, hydrogenated fats or oils
- ○ Caffeine (too much)

Foods Lower Cortisol Levels:

Many natural whole foods offer health benefits and essential nutrients. For example, increasing your intake of vitamin C, which is found in citrus fruits such as oranges, as well as some vegetables including bell peppers and dark green leafy vegetables, can reduce negative high cortisol side effects. When cortisol levels are high add these to your diet:

- **Water**

  - ○ is the most neutralizing substance on the planet, water can flush excess cortisol out of the body before it can cause damage and studies show dehydration increases cortisol buildup in the body.

- **Dark Chocolate**

  - ○ Two studies showed that consuming dark chocolate reduces the cortisol response.

- **Fruits**

  - ○ Eating bananas or pears reduces cortisol levels.

- **Black and Green Tea**

  - ○ Studies show drinking black tea decreased cortisol

- **Probiotics and Prebiotics**

  - ○ Prebiotics provide food for good bacteria to grow. Such as:

    - ■ soluble fiber

  - ○ Probiotics are friendly, symbiotic bacteria. Both probiotics and prebiotics help reduce cortisol so consuming these foods help:

- Yogurt (plain or plant based)
- Sauerkraut
- Kimchi

Some Negative Health Results of Having High Cortisol are:

- High Inflammation
- Adrenal Depletion
- High Blood Pressure
- Accelerated Aging
- and more

Foods high in omega-3 fatty acids may also help with the other side effects of high cortisol such as inflammation caused by high cortisol. Some of the cortisol lowering foods are:

- Halibut
- Walnuts
- Almonds
- Flaxseed Oil
- Vitamin C

The bottom line is that over time, a bad lifestyle that triggers continual high cortisol levels can accelerate aging, lead to weight gain, high blood pressure, diabetes, fatigue, difficulty concentrating, poor health, misery, suffering and eventually, early death.

Chapter 3

Your Metabolism & Metabolic System

Metabolic System

Your main metabolic organ is your Liver. The metabolic activities of the liver are essential for providing fuel to the brain, muscle, and other peripheral organs.

Liver's Job

The liver produces over 500,000 enzymes each day to maintain its normal metabolic functions.

Toxins Stress Liver And Metabolism

Toxic substances such as hydrogenated cooking oils rob the liver of its metabolic enzymes, it takes 51 days to metabolise one molecule of hydrogenated fat.

The liver is a large organ and can be from 2% to 4% of your body weight. Other metabolic organs are:

- Liver
- Adrenals
- Thyroid
- Pituitary
- Pancreas
- Brain
- Muscle
- Adipose Tissue
- Kidney

Metabolism is the process by which your body converts what you eat and drink into energy. During this complex biochemical process, calories in food and beverages arc combined with oxygen to release the energy your body needs to function. The word metabolism can also refer to the sum of all chemical reactions that occur in living organisms, including digestion and the transport of substances into and between different cells, in which case the above described set of reactions within the cells is called intermediary metabolism or intermediate metabolism.

Metabolic reactions may be categorized as:

- Catabolic- is the breaking down of compounds (for example, the breaking down glucose to pyruvate by cellular respiration
- Anabolic- is the building up or synthesis proteins, carbohydrates, lipids, and nucleic acids.
- Catabolism releases energy.
- Anabolism consumes energy.

Your most important metabolic pathways are:

- Glycolysis glucose oxidation in order to obtain ATP.
- Acetyl-CoA oxidation in order to obtain GTP and intermediates.
- Oxidative phosphorylation - disposal of the electrons released by glycolysis and citric acid cycle.

Digestive Enzymes & Metabolism

Virtually all living things, including those we cook and eat, contain enzymes. In fact there are over 3000 different kinds of enzymes. The raw foods are rich with enzymes which help us digest them and help our digestive track break down, assimilate and utilize nutrition during metabolism. Plants, fruits and vegetables contain active enzymes. Upon eating raw spinach, the cells of the leaf are immediately broken down, successfully releasing its nutrients. Mother's milk too has a host of enzymes that are valuable in infant digestion and the production of good bacteria. In fact all living animals produce enzymes in their digestive tract. Enzymes are so indispensable that they are often described as the spark plugs for the vast majority of chemical reactions that make life possible.

The public has been well-versed on digestive enzymes, and they are commonly taken as dietary supplements. Digestive enzymes have been long recognized for their importance in the digestive process.

Systemic Enzymes & Aging Tissues

Systemic enzymes digest excess metabolic waste, inflammation and fibrin in the body. Fibrin is a fibrillar protein that creates scar tissue and fibrin is the main component that is responsible for the unhealthy build-up of scar tissue, arterial plaque, toxins, viruses, thrombus formation as well as the spider web of tissue that tend to encase our internal organs with age. Enzymes can prevent fibrin from being deposited in wounds forming scar tissue, fractures and joints. Systemic enzymes also remove necrotic debris and excess fibrin from the bloodstream. Proteolytic enzymes are used in enzyme therapy to dissolve fibrin. When strong proteolytic enzymes are taken as a therapeutic enzyme preparation as an alternative for scar tissue surgery. In Germany, every surgical patient is given systemic enzymes before surgery to prevent blood clots and scar tissue. Enzymes can be powerful enough to gradually digest scar tissue away. This takes time to occur, of course, but eventually all the scar tissue should disappear.

Metabolic And Hormone Balance Disruptors

To keep these two bodily systems in balance it is important to limit your exposure to toxins and endocrine system disruptors. The worst enemies to our health and longevity are:

1. Environmental toxins
2. Food toxins
3. Water toxins
4. Air toxins
5. Stress hormones (cortisol in combination with toxins)
6. Cardio exercise does not burn fat it does the opposite.
7. Medium paced exercise burns fat boost metabolism
8. Short burst high-intensity stimulates anti-aging mechanisms.

Silent Age Accelerators

In modern society, there are hidden toxins in many places, from breathing smog living in cities to living in water damaged buildings riddled with mold mycotoxins or eating a diet of processed foods that are heavy laden with preservatives, artificial flavors and food dyes and colors and drinking artificial drinks which are chemical compounds and when all these compounds are mixed with other chemicals in unison our environmental health becomes no longer safe. Some food additives may be safe in small one-serving doses but in combination with other chemicals or environmental pollutants such as smog, pesticides, herbicides and nitrate fertilizers, it can become a deadly cocktail. The more toxic the environment and the more processed the food the greater the burden is on the body's state of homeostasis and the metabolism. The body is intended to metabolise foods in their natural state, only.

Body's 1ˢᵗ Overload

The liver must produce over 500,000 enzymes a day just to regulate normal metabolic functions. Add a load of toxins and the liver can't keep up with eliminating the body of toxins and a build up of toxins occur. Toxic overload is when the body systems can no longer keep up with eliminating the toxins because the overload has stressed the eliminative organ systems beyond their capacity. The digestive system, immune system, hormone system and biochemical systems begin to malfunction and then disease states set in and begin to develop. All of the bodily systems need to maintain balance to function properly and the more natural your diet and environment is, the better your body is able to maintain good health and proper functioning and the longer and healthier your life will be.

Environmental Toxins Age Us

Smoke, UV rays, pollution, heavy metals and other toxins in our environment can introduce free radicals in the body, in essence fueling the processes behind oxidative stress. Toxins cause chronic inflammation which is a result of oxidative stress among other causes but, all of these factors can potentially speed up the aging process.

What Your Body Needs To Live A Long Life

The body needs clean nourishment and a safe environment to stay healthy and in a state of function that is conducive to longevity. The body's basic necessities are:

1. Clean Air
2. Clean Food
3. Clean Water
4. Clean Shelter
5. Low Stress Hormone Activation

Stress Age Accelerator

Cortisol is the stress hormone and it blocks your testosterone levels and high levels of cortisol inhibits the testosterone function leading to sluggish metabolism, low sex drive, weight gain and lowered motivation. When cortisol levels are high it blocks testosterone metabolism and it can increase dihydrotestosterone.

- Lose muscle mass
- Gain Weight
- Increase cardiovascular heart problems
- Increase Ab, Hip and Thigh Fat
- Irritable Mood
- Trouble Sleeping
- Hair on the Face
- Male Pattern Baldness

Borderline Hormone Imbalance

The adrenal glands produce cortisol and in women the adrenals also begin to produce testosterone in women around menopause. 99% of the time the "middle age spread" is caused by a borderline hormonal imbalance. In other words, the hormones are within what is considered to be the normal range, yet still the person experiences all the symptoms of a hormone imbalance. For example, your estrogen levels were on the low end of normal range and your testosterone level may be on the high end of normal range, even though both are within the range of normal it causes age related symptoms associated with menopause in women and in reverse, andropause in men. The medical approach to treatment is to do nothing until the hormones are completely out of balance. However, if you are in a borderline range it is important to take preventative action to correct it before you develop hormones that go out of normal range.

Chapter 4
Preventing Hormonal Imbalances

Hormones are specialized chemicals that carry messages from the endocrine glands where they're produced to organs and cells throughout your body. Hormones influence nearly every bodily function from digestion and fat-burning to mood and cognition. Hormones affect specific organs and cells in your body, but they also interact with each other to regulate and compensate for one another. Because your body and its relationship with hormones is complex, a small imbalance can adversely impact your health. Therefore, learning to recognize the signs of hormone imbalances can help ensure that you recognize the early signs so you stay healthy.

Examples Of Hormones:

- Cortisol - stress hormone
- Adrenaline - fight or flight hormone
- Estrogen - female sex hormone
- Testosterone - male sex hormone
- Insulin - regulates normal blood sugar levels
- Glucagon - hepatic glucose production
- T4 - a thyroid hormone
- T3 - a thyroid hormone

Hormones control your:

- Mood
- appetite,
- blood sugar,
- energy levels,
- stress response,
- sleep schedule,
- sex drive,

- sexual function,
- fertility.

In fact, hormones influence nearly every bodily function from digestion and fat-burning to mood and cognition.

Hormones affect specific organs and cells in your body, but they also affect one another. Because your body and its relationship with hormones is complex, a small imbalance can adversely impact your health. Therefore, learning to recognize the signs of hormone imbalances can help ensure you stay healthy.

Signs of Hormone Imbalance

Here's a list of signs and symptoms that indicate a hormone imbalance in women:

- Sleep issues
- Fatigue or tiredness
- Reliance on caffeine to get through the day
- Poor memory or concentration
- Mood problems (irritability, depression, or anxiety)
- Appetite changes
- Weight gain or loss
- Sugar or carbohydrate cravings
- Becoming "hangry" (angry when hungry)
- Temperature sensitivity
- Facial hair
- Low libido
- Erratic sex drive
- Bloating or water retention
- Enlarged or tender breasts
- Aches and pains
- Irregular menstrual cycles
- Heavy or prolonged bleeding
- Hot flashes
- Vaginal dryness
- Infertility
- Headaches
- High blood pressure
- Rapid heart rate

These are some of the typical symptoms indicating that you may have a hormone imbalance. However, you can fix your hormone levels and reduce the symptoms of hormone imbalances. You don't have to live with tiredness, mood issues, or low libido.

Best Supplements for Balancing Your Hormones

Every hormone imbalance is slightly different–therefore, you should experiment with lifestyle changes, including health supplements, to see what works best for your situation.

Hormone Balancing For Anti-Aging

DIM is the best compound to balance and stabilize all hormone imbalances. DIM also reverses Nrf2 gene silencing in transgenic mice with prostate cancer tissues, inducing Nrf2 expression, and subsequently, NQO1 expression to help prevent cancer.

DIM The Ultimate Hormone Balancer

Diindolylmethane (DIM) is a phytochemical from cruciferous vegetables, Some cruciferous vegetables are broccoli, kale, watercress and cabbage. In your digestive tract, cruciferous vegetables break down into indole-3-carbinol and convert into DIM during digestion. DIM balances and stabilizes the entire endocrine system and all of the hormones it produces, especially, estrogen. DIM also inhibits aromatase which is the enzyme that converts testosterone into estrogen. Lastly, DIM partially blocks the effect of dihydrotestosterone, a bad residue that leads to signs of aging such as male pattern baldness and enlarged prostate gland. Research also shows DIM (diindolylmethane) helps:

- Lower bad estrogen
- Lower Cancer risk (some)

    o breast & prostate cancer.

- Lower obesity
- Reduce inflammation
- Increase Cognitive Function
- Neuroprotective

DIM is beneficial for providing you a healthier functioning body and it is safe, too. Animal safety studies show that even a dose of DIM ten times greater than therapeutic doses is not dangerous.

DHEA

DHEA (dehydroepiandrosterone) supplementation is safe in small doses and improves quality of life in those showing signs of aging.

DHEA is a so-called precursor hormone to many hormones that decline with age. DHEA is converted by the body to estrogens and androgens, it is also a precursor to testosterone. It is possible that supplementation with DHEA may increase estrogen and testosterone levels in peri-andropausal men and peri- and postmenopausal women to decrease hormone decline symptoms and improve general wellbeing and sexual function in both men and women. During menopause a fluctuation and eventually a decrease in estrogen levels occur. DHEA helps improve:

- Hormonal changes
- Andropause & menopausal symptoms
- Hot flashes
- Night sweats
- Irritability
- Mood swings (hormonal)

Hormone Supporting Anti-Aging Supplements

- **Melatonin**

    Melatonin, also called the 'sleep hormone' is a hormone produced by the body to regulate the sleep cycle. However, it has now been determined to have age reversing properties too. Melatonin effective for reverse aging is that it scavenges free radicals from the body and prevents them from harming healthy cells in the body tissues. As the body gets more prone to disease and mutation with age, the chances of free radicals exerting harmful effects also increases. Melatonin supplements can help reduce this probability. It is said to act on a cellular level, working on DNA to guard it against disease and illnesses that come with age. It helps in protecting various body organs and helps delay the onset of various diseases like adult onset diabetes.

- **DHEA Testosterone Booster**

    DHEA is both a natural hormone and popular supplement that can affect the levels of other hormones in your body such as testosterone. It has been studied for its potential to increase bone density, decrease body fat, improve sexual function and correct some hormonal problems. Testosterone is a steroid hormone produced by the body in both males and females. In females it is produced in negligible amounts, whereas in males, it is produced in greater amounts. DHEA is necessary for the development of their secondary sexual characteristics. For men, testosterone supplements can help a lot with reverse aging. It affects their overall wellbeing and its increased levels, same as those in their youth and helps feel them younger. It keeps a man's energy level and sex drive high and greater muscle mass. A number of studies have found that DHEA supplements may help people with depression, obesity, lupus, and adrenal insufficiency. DHEA may also improve skin in older people and help treat osteoporosis, vaginal atrophy, erectile dysfunction, and some psychological conditions. Melatonin and DHEA interact to control production of the other. When melatonin is highest, NREM sleep occurs; when DHEA increases slightly during sleep to maintain brainstem function, REM sleep occurs. During sleep, DHEA is low to reduce stimulation of the CNS, so sleep may occur.

- **Estrogen and Progesterone**

    Estrogen and progesterone are female steroid hormones. They are also produced by the male body, but in negligible amounts. All women start feeling the effects well before their menopause, be it hot flashes or mood swings. Even the very thought of their approaching menopausal period is enough for women to genuinely get depressed that they are aging.

    Estrogen and progesterone can help with specific aging issues. These hormones help women maintain their sexual drive, physical and mental wellbeing and an overall youthful appearance. Various plants and herbs have very high contents of estrogen. When these are incorporated in diet, they can have age defying effects. However, estrogen supplements are also easily available and are completely safe, given they are not taken excessively.

DHT Blocker

Dihydrotestosterone (DHT) can contribute to many age related conditions in the body, from an enlarged prostate to hair loss, baldness and even poses an elevated risk factor for cancer in men and additionally, female hormonal imbalances and thinning, brittle hair loss in women. Using DHT blockers may help return your DHT levels to normal and allow your hair to regrow.

Best Natural DHT Blocker Foods:

- Caffeine applied topically to scalp
- Green tea
- Saw palmetto
- Pygeum
- Stinging nettle
- Fcnugreek
- Soy
- Pumpkin seed oil
- Tea tree oil
- Lycopene Foods

    o Tomato
    o Grapefruit
    o Apricot
    o Pink guava
    o Watermelon

Chasteberry - Sex Hormone Balance

Chasteberry- an extract from the chaste tree known as vitex agnus or monk's pepper tree that is native to the Mediterranean region of Europe, is a good hormone balancer. Research of chasteberry shows that one of the ways chasteberry works is by enhancing the function of the neurotransmitter dopamine. However, its other mechanisms of action aren't currently well understood.

Women have long used Chasteberry supplements to ease PMS pain of their menstrual cycles and to help improve mood and others report they have had success with improvement of infertility for both men and women. Chasteberry may help prevent:

- Oxidative stress,
- Nutritional deficiencies,
- Hormone balance
- Anti-aging

Chasteberry is also helpful for many other symptoms related to aging. However, it is not recommended for pregnant or nursing women to take it as there is no evidence that it is 100% safe during pregnancy.

Maca for Sexual Function Healthy Hormones

Maca root, also called Peruvian ginseng, is an edible plant from Peru. Research shows that maca root enhances serum levels of luteinizing hormone, enhances fertility. Maca is consumed fresh, cooked as a root vegetable or it can be ground into a flour for making bread or smoothies. For early postmenopausal women, maca can increase bone density, improve the hormonal processes of the reproductive axis, balance hormone levels, relieve symptoms such as hot flashes or night sweats and maca helps reduce the need for hormone replacement therapy (HRT)Maca can also help reduce blood pressure and improve symptoms of depression in menopausal women.

- Better Moods
- Energy & Stamina
- Hormonal Health Improvement
- Reduced Altitude Sickness
- Reduce Anxiety

A study of men given a maca root daily for four months found that the treatment increased their seminal volume, sperm count, motile sperm count, and sperm motility, but did not alter their hormone levels and men given maca root daily for three months increased their libido increased.

Probiotics for Mood and Gut Health

Probiotics are good bacteria, it is the natural occurring bacteria found in your digestive tract. It is very important to your health as the bacteria in your gut help comprise your microbiome. The health of your microbiome affects your:

- metabolism,
- digestion,
- neurotransmitter production.

Common things that can wipe out your beneficial bacteria within your microbiome are:

- Poor diet,

- inflammation, and the
- use of antibiotics

In order to repopulate your gut with good bacteria and probiotics, you should eat an anti-inflammatory diet:

- Avoid antibiotic laced commercial foods
- Eat organic produce
- Eat growth hormone free foods, eggs and dairy
- Take a probiotic supplement.

Probiotic bacteria help your body produce serotonin and other neurotransmitters, probiotic supplements can be helpful for people with:

- depression,
- anxiety, and
- other mood disorders.

An overgrowth of harmful gut bacteria can cause your health to deteriorate and by taking probiotics you can help stabilize your gut with the good bacteria and enhance your immune function.

Ascorbic Acid For Better Immune Function

Vitamin C is an essential nutrient and antioxidant involved in tissue repair and enzymatic production of neurotransmitters. It helps your body absorb iron and is also required for immune function.

Vitamin C supplementation can reduce:

- Free radical damage
- Stress hormones and cortisol
- Adrenaline levels.

Vitamin C can also improve:

- Immune function,
- Reduce oxidative stress, and
- Lower inflammation in your body
- Reduce high blood pressure and

- Neutralize other negative effects of stress,
- Lowers anxiety hormones
- Lowers fasting blood glucose
- Reduces the risk of gestational diabetes mellitus
- Reduces inflammation and periodontal disease
- Helps reverse motor and cognitive impairments
- Helps symptoms of dementia
- Helps symptoms of neurodegenerative conditions
- Lowers cancer risk

Fruits Rich in Vitamin C:

- Citrus
- Orange,
- Kiwi,
- Lemon,
- Guava,
- Grapefruit,
- Papaya,
- Cantaloupe
- Strawberries.

Vegetables Rich in Vitamin C:

- Broccoli, Brussels sprouts, and cauliflower.
- Green and red peppers.
- Spinach,
- Cabbage,
- Turnip greens,
- Leafy greens.
- Sweet and white potatoes.
- Tomatoes
- Winter squash.

Magnesium Your Body's Superconductor

Magnesium is an essential mineral that is key to the function of over 300 enzymes that regulate most bodily functions and additionally, it is used in many more physiological processes. Taking magnesium supplements can mitigate the effects of stress, reduce inflammation, improve your sleep, normalize your heart rhythms, and lower your blood pressure. Additionally, magnesium paired with vitamin B6 is more effective to reduce severe stress than magnesium alone.

Magnesium can reduce:

- Stress and
- Anxiety and improve severe
- PMS symptoms

Magnesium Deficiency Symptoms

Even if you eat a healthy diet, most people do not get enough magnesium from food because of magnesium stripping food processing and environmental factors.

Magnesium deficiency can result in:

- high blood pressure
- poor sleep
- irregular heartbeat.

Magnesium Rich Foods:

- Figs
- Almonds
- Cashews
- Pumpkin Seeds
- Spinach
- Peanuts
- Avocados
- Guavas
- Bananas
- Kiwi fruit
- Papayas
- Blackberries
- Raspberries
- Cantaloupes
- Grapefruit

Zinc Aging And Immunity

Zinc is an essential mineral required in your body for the function or production of over 1000 transcription factors. It is the second most abundant trace metal in humans next to iron. Zinc can help:

- Prevent grey hair,
- Increase libido and
- Enhance brain function and
- Balance emotional health.

Adding more zinc to your diet may boost your mood and keep you from feeling depressed and resist the effects of stress. After menopause, supplementing with zinc may help improve bone mass.

Zinc Deficiency

Low levels of zinc can originate from poor diet but also from aging and factors like disease. Being vegetarian may also increase your risk of zinc deficiency.

Copper Anti-Aging Super Star

Copper is an essential mineral and anti-aging miracle. It plays diverse roles in biological electron transport as well as the transportation of oxygen. Your body also uses copper to make the antioxidant superoxide dismutase. Superoxide dismutase prevents cell damage in your body that would otherwise be caused by free radicals. If you take copper supplements, you may be less likely to get depressed. During pregnancy, copper intake may also help eliminate morning sickness. Taking copper may help prevent osteoporosis and fractures. Copper supplements can also reverse heart enlargement caused by pressure overload].

Copper Deficiency

Deficiencies of copper can produce symptoms similar to anemia including:

- Bone abnormalities
- Impaired growth
- Infections
- Osteoporosis
- Disrupted glucose and
- Cholesterol metabolism.

- Heart disease

Excess alcohol consumption may result in copper deficiency.

Calcium for Chemistry Balance & Bone Health

Calcium is an essential mineral and there are over a quarter of a million types of calcium. Various types of calcium have various effects in the body. Some types of calcium keep your body chemistry alkalized, some aid muscle actions, some build strong teeth and bone and some are used for other functions in the body. As we age and sex hormone levels decrease, the risk of muscle weakness, bone loss and other problems and issues calcium loss increases. Calcium supplements can help prevent age related muscle strength and bone loss and improve your bone density. As you age, supplementing with calcium as well as getting twenty minutes of sun exposure for vitamin D production can improve your mood, strength and also reduce your risk of bone fractures and improve your agility from falling or other accidents.

Calcium Deficiency

Calcium needs increase during menstrual cycles but both men and women can have symptoms such as:

- Muscle Cramps
- Sore Muscles
- Pain
- Constipation

Glycine for Sleep and Anxiety

Glycine is a nonessential amino acid and inhibitory neurotransmitter found in your central nervous system. Taking glycine before bedtime can improve subjective and objective sleep quality in people who struggle with insomnia. Glycine before bed reduces:

- Next-morning fatigue,
- Enhances sleep satisfaction,
- Increases sleep efficiency, and
- Reduces the difficulty of sleep onset.
- Reduces core body temperature,
- Increases health and well-being by

- Reverses symptoms of metabolic disorders,
- Relieves cardiovascular diseases,
- Inflammatory diseases,
- Obesity,
- Diabetes
- Cancer
- Schizophrenia

When glycine levels in your body are low, your body may make less glutathione. Glutathione is an antioxidant that is vital for your body's proper functioning. Boosting cellular glutathione levels by obtaining more glycine through diet and supplements may help prevent and treat disorders caused by oxidative stress.

Hormone Summary

Your hormones affect your overall health in significant ways. Stress, mood, libido, PMS, and the severity of menopausal symptoms can all be influenced by your hormone levels. Your endocrine system is complex, but you can use natural supplements and other lifestyle changes to improve your hormonal health. However, if you are suffering from severe hormone imbalance symptoms, you should speak to an endocrinologist or other trusted healthcare practitioner.

The benefits of balancing your hormones include reduced cravings, better blood sugar levels, greater energy, less stress, and improved fertility.

Why We Need Testosterone

When Cortisol is Balanced And Testosterone Levels are good.

- Better Memory
- Healthy Weight
- Better Bone
- Better Sex Drive

What to do to improve testosterone level naturally:

- Lower stress
- Take an adrenal boosting adaptogen supplement
- Add Cortisol Lowering Foods To Your Diet:

- o Pine Pollen
- o Tribulus

Cortisol Lowering Testosterone Boosting Plants:

- **Pine Pollen**
  Pine pollen can lower high cortisol levels up to 25%. It can also elevate testosterone levels, naturally.

- **Saw Palmetto**
  Saw palmetto is an extract from the berries of a palmetto palm tree.

  - o Helps prevent graying of the hair
  - o Ease age related urinary continence
  - o Helps improve prostate health

- **Pygeum**
  A human study of pygeum extract did not find significant changes in testosterone, follicle-stimulating hormone, luteinizing hormone, or estrogens. Pygeum is from a tree bark, it is used as medicine.

Pygeum is used for treating symptoms of:

- increase sexual desire
- enlarged prostate
- benign prostatic hyperplasia, BPH
- prostate cancer.

Pygeum is also used for:

- pain caused by inflammation,
- kidney disease,
- urinary problems,
- malaria,
- stomachache,
- fever.

- **Long Jack**
  Tongkat ali or longjack, is an herbal supplement that comes from the roots of the green shrub tree Eurycoma longifolia plant.

- ○ increases testosterone in men and women
- ○ erectile dysfunction,
- ○ increasing sexual desire,
- ○ male infertility, and
- ○ boosting energy and athletic performance

- **Tribulus Terrestris**
  Is a fruit-producing Mediterranean plant. The steroid saponins of tribulus terrestris have a stimulating effect on both male and female sexual function.

  - Tribulus can cause as much as a 50% increase testosterone
  - Tribulus lowers Cortisol the stress hormone.
  - Helps improve gains in strength
  - Leaner muscle mass in 5-28 days.

- **Hawthorne**
  Hawthorn berry contains plant polyphenols that have been linked to numerous health benefits due to their antioxidant properties and polyphenols and offers numerous health benefits, including a lower risk of the following

  - Cancer (some types)
  - Diabetes (type 2)
  - Asthma
  - Infections (some types)
  - Heart problems (some types)
  - Skin aging (premature)

- **Chrysin**
  Crysin occurs naturally in various plants and substances, such as the passionflower. Lowers cortisol it is found in foods such as honey and propolis and can reduce bad estrogens. Chrysin is an aromatase inhibitor. It is in a subgroup of phytochemicals that can inhibit the proliferation of cancer cells.

- **Horny Goat Weed**
  A flowering herbal plant that is a key herb in Chinese medicine for low libido, it also helps with:

  - Erectile dysfunction
  - Helps prevent osteoporosis
  - Sexual dysfunction (male or female)

■ Menopausal symptoms

Future Technology Anti-Aging

Xenobots Tiny 'xenobots' assembled from cells promise advances for better health, from drug delivery to toxic waste clean-up.

Systemic Enzymes

Systemic enzymes help to speed the resolution of fibrin, clear out cellular waste from the blood to support normal liver function and boost the immune system. There are many types of systemic enzymes one example is the systemic enzyme, serratiopeptidase, has anti-inflammatory properties and is used to supplement the diet for this benefit.

Worldwide Life Span Extension

The estimated "natural" life span of humans have extended to beyond 80 years in most developed countries. However, much of the population now experiences aging-associated tissue deterioration. Healthy aging is limited by a lack of natural selection, which favors genetic programs that confer fitness early in life to maximize reproductive output. There is no selection for whether these alterations have detrimental effects later in life. One such program is cellular senescence, whereby cells become unable to divide.

Cellular senescence enhances reproductive success by blocking cancer cell proliferation, but it decreases the health of the old by littering tissues with dysfunctional senescent cells (SNCs). In mice, the selective elimination of SNCs extends median life span and prevents or attenuates age-associated diseases. This has inspired the development of targeted senolytic drugs to eliminate the SNCs that drive age-associated disease in humans.

Chapter 5

Sirtuins, Genes, Telomeres & DNA

Your genes do play a major role in your health. Sirtuins can turn on and off genes but as we age the telomeres shorten until we die. The good news is, if you take good care of your genes you can save yourself from developing most adult onset illnesses even if you have a genetic predisposition for particular diseases by hereditary factors.

Good Gene's

Genetics aren't the only thing at play in longevity. Genome, nutrition, fitness and ethnicity are intertwined together and we are just now uncovering some of the secrets encoded in the human genome. The genome is evolving constantly via epigenetics. Every individual has his or her own distinct genome. The ethnic relationship, genomic stability and genetic distribution are all real and have significant long term impacts on our genome and in turn on human evolution. There are several natural substances that you can take to help turn back and slow down the hands of time on your age clock as you will discover as you read this book.

The Klotho Gene Is Closely Associated To Anti-Aging Functions In Mammals

Support Your Genes

You can have a positive impact on your genes! Supporting telomcre / DNA can help you boost your cell function. Without proper support, cells become less healthy and can stop replicating and die. Naturally boost your cell's ability to support your body in all of its functions. DNA and RNA enable the correct identification of invaders to trigger immune function offering vital immune support.

- **Omega Fatty Acids**

  Fish oils are the best source of omega-3 and omega-6 fatty acids. These have natural anti-inflammatory properties that play a vital role in any anti-aging regime. These omegas help the body in regulating its various functions, including blood pressure, maintenance of body temperature and proper functioning of the heart. Omega fatty acids essentially help keep the heart young by ensuring that it is strong enough to function properly and prevent the clotting of blood under normal circumstances. Infact, fish oil supplements are also advised by physicians to heart patients, for prevention of any further cardiac problems. But the benefits don't stop there. Fish oils also have a significant anti-aging impact on the brain. They prevent the development of brain diseases and also help the brain maintain its thinking abilities, which normally reduces with growing age. Fish oils have also been found to protect against dementia and other memory related disorders. Fish oil capsules can take off years from your face too. They help healthy skin cells live longer and reduce the probability of damage to these cells, keeping the skin vibrant and youthful.

- **Alpha Lipoic Acid**

  Alpha lipoic acid supplements can be very helpful when you want to stop the signs of aging. Alpha lipoic acid also has antioxidant properties that find and destroy free radicals in the body. The antioxidant property of alpha lipoic acid is more potent than of other supplements because it destroys free radicals from any part of the body. Alpha lipoic acid can cross the blood brain barrier, exerting its effects on the brain and protecting against age related diseases like dementia. Another effect that makes it ideal for reverse aging is that it lengthens telomeres. By supplementing with alpha lipoic acid, you can ensure that your telomeres stay in optimal health and delay the onset of premature aging.

- **Astragalus**

  A very common herb used in natural medicine for its immune boosting properties additionally offers anti-aging benefits as certain astragalus molecules have been found to contribute to telomere growth. Telomeres are parts on DNA strands directly responsible for cellular aging which acts as protective caps at the end of each DNA strand without which the strands would become damaged and the cells would no longer able to do their job properly. Telomeres have the tendency to shorten as an individual ages. Eventually they may become too short to do their job properly and cause the cells to age. So, essentially longer telomeres are markers of healthy cells while shorter ones are connected to premature cellular aging. Astragalus, increased telomerase activity.

- **Resveratrol**

  Resveratrol is a compound naturally found in grapes and nuts. The age reversing properties are not limited to just skin alone but may help keep age related disorders at bay as well. The primary mechanism by which resveratrol does this is by acting on a group of enzymes called sirtuins. Sirtuins are enzymes that affect various metabolic pathways of the human body that are involved in the aging process. Research has shown resveratrol stimulating these proteins directly, increasing mitochondrial activity which results in producing energy within the cells. This, in turn, can have the effect of extending cellular life. Also, being a naturally occurring type of antibiotic, resveratrol can work to cleanse the body of pollutants and other contaminants. Among other things, this action is also beneficial for keeping the skin healthier, fresher, and youthful. The same can also prevent future wrinkles and reduce the appearance of existing ones. The resveratrol in most supplements comes from knotweed.

- **Resveratrol**- is one of the anti-aging compounds such as antioxidants and polyphenols that is in grapes or wine. You can take a supplement without drinking wine.

  Resveratrol is in common foods such as:

  - grapes,
  - peanuts,
  - cocoa,
  - pistachios,
  - wine,
  - cranberries,
  - blueberries
  - dark chocolate.

Many plants make resveratrol to fight fungal infections, UV injury, radiation and stress.

Researchers in genetics have discovered that resveratrol can:

- increase cell survival
- slow aging
- activate the "longevity" gene sirtuin one (SIRT1)

Resveratrol can help:

- prevent skin cancer
- protect against:

  - high blood pressure
  - heart failure
  - heart disease

- improve insulin sensitivity
- reduce blood sugar
- blunt obesity induced by a high-fat diet

- **Hyaluronic Acid**

  Hyaluronic acid is a naturally occurring substance found in the skin that keeps the skin looking young and makes it glow. It works primarily by helping the skin retain moisture and stay well hydrated. This ensures that all the extra water you are drinking to keep your skin healthy, stays within the skin. With age, the skin automatically loses its ability to retain water, losing hydration and elasticity. This increases wrinkles and fine lines on the face. Hyaluronic acid slows down this process to a great degree, keeping the skin firm and supple.

Fisetin Stops Damaged DNA From Replicating

Fisetin is a plant polyphenol from the flavonoid group of nutrients. Fisetin is an anti-aging compound and like other polyphenols such as resveratrol but it is a sirtuin-activating compound that has been shown in laboratory studies to extend the lifespan. According to studies published by the NIH National Institutes researchers,

Fisetin The Great Protector Of Your Inner Fountain Of Youth

Fisetin is a senotherapeutic. Fisetin extends health and lifespan. Senescence is a tumor suppressor mechanism that is activated in stressed cells to prevent replication of damaged DNA. Senescent cells have been demonstrated to play a causal role in driving aging and age-related diseases. Both, fisetin and the flavonoid quercetin are potent senolytics that may help in improving numerous age-related conditions including age related frailty, osteoporosis and cardiovascular disease. Fisetin has also shown anti-cancer activity in studies on cells.

- Fisetin
- Quercetin

Effects Of Telomere Loss

The telomere-shortening process is a leading contributor to physiologic and pathophysiologic changes that occur with aging. At a critical point, telomeres lose their protective capacity and at this point senescence signaling is initiated. This process is central to the pathogenesis of many cardiovascular conditions. As for the longevity genes, these are a subset of genes identified to have a major role in aging.

- catalase and insulin-like growth factor 1; others include:
- the sirtuins,
- forkhead box transcription factors,
- pituitary-specific positive class 1 homeobox

The name for the *"klotho-gene"* came from Clotho the goddess who spins the thread of life in Greek mythology. Klotho is an anti-aging protein compound that is mainly secreted by your kidneys, your brain and also by your thyroid. Klotho plays a major role in regulating your kidney function and your vascular health.

Klotho Upregulation By Rapamycin Protects Against Vascular Disease

Additionally, Aerobic exercise-stimulated Klotho upregulation extends life span by attenuating the excess production of reactive oxygen species in the brain a subset of the longevity genes interacts extensively to regulate processes that determine age-associated physiological adaptations and some of those are.

- mitochondrial function,
- stress response,
- metabolism
- age-associated physiological adaptations
- many other age-associated processes

For example, the roles of oxidative stress in the onset of age-related cardiovascular disease and the involvement of telomeres, longevity genes and the longevity network are age-related cardiovascular disorders that are activated in response to oxidative stress based challenges.

DNA Methylation Age Test

DNA methylation is bad because just as high homocysteine can be damaging to your blood vessels, methylation can have the same effect in the brain by damaging your neurons and causing inflammation which lead to deterioration of cognitive function and the onset of dementia, alzhimers and other age related mental decline issues. Multiple studies have linked poor methylation to cognitive problems. The key to anti-aging is by utilizing methods of turning back your biological clock, which is regulated by methylation.

Horvath Clock Test

Horvath's epigenetic clock was developed by professor Steve Horvath, a professor in human genetics and biostatistics at UCLA. Dr. Horvath spent over 4 years collecting publicly available Illumina DNA methylation data and identifying statistical methods to measure a person's age based on their DNA Methylation.

Epigenome

The Epigenome is what allows us all to develop into a fully developed human being. Proteins spool up, switch off genes and as we age there is a loss of analog information in DNA replication.

Avoid DNA Breaks

Broken chromosomes lose their cellular identity and the outcome is aging. Unless there is good medical reason avoid radiation, MRI's, CT Scans unless you are having symptoms which require these types of exposures as according to research experts, as these types of test potentially damage and break your DNA. In Mice studies, those who had DNA breaks aged +50%. However, it is important to monitor your health, so go to your doctor and have a blood test or have your genome sequenced. It is better to get a blood test

NMN (Nicotinamide)

Switches on energy genes, stamina, youthful ability for a person's optimal physical performance, it's the high octane fuel for the body. NMN and hunger work the same aging pathways.

NMN Age Reversal

Nicotinamide mononucleotide (NMN) is a nucleotide derived from ribose and nicotinamide. NMN is made from B vitamins in the body or by supplementation with NMN, a precursor of NAD+ which has been shown to improve metabolism and reduce aging markers while increasing sirtuin activity. At Harvard university research center, the first long-term lifespan study in mice involving supplementation with NMN, a precursor of NAD+ metabolism, was shown to reduce aging markers and increase sirtuin activity. One way cells manufacture NAD begins with a precursor molecule called nicotinamide mononucleotide (NMN), which is found naturally in foods such as:

- Avocado
- Brussel sprouts
- Broccoli
- Cabbage
- Cucumber
- Edamame

Research found that NMN elevates NAD+ levels in cells throughout the body and is better absorbed than taking NAD as a supplement. Nicotinamide adenine dinucleotide is a cofactor central to metabolism. NAD is found in all living cells. We need energy to exercise, so establishing a regular fitness routine stimulates mitochondria production and naturally boosts your NAD+ levels. To improve NAD in the body.

- Fast for Faster Metabolism
- Protect Your Body From Too Much Sunlight
- Take NAD-Infused Supplements
- Eat A NAD Rich Diet
- Make Sure You Get Enough Sleep

Empower Your Metabolism To Make New Cells

There are some newly discovered compounds that are critical to power metabolism, construct new cellular components, mitochondrial regeneration, resist free radical and DNA damage:

- Nicotinamide mononucleotide (NMN) (precursor to NAD)
- Nicotinamide Adenine Dinucleotide (NAD plus) NAD+

Research has found that NAD+ dramatically improves anti-aging by enhancing longevity sirtuin gene expression. When we boost NMN levels in the body, we can enhance the natural biosynthesis of NAD+ and alleviate symptoms associated with age-related degeneration.

- Healthy mitochondrial function is an important component of healthy human aging. Our body naturally has the ability to make NAD+ from the food we eat. As we age, levels of NAD+ decline substantially. This decline leaves us at greater risk for neuro and muscular degeneration declines our cardio-metabolic health and our capacity for repair
- Clinical studies led by Dr. David Sinclair at Harvard University suggest that boosting NAD+ using NMN is key to increasing the amount of time we spend in good health. NAD+ is a relatively unstable compound and cannot be taken orally as a supplement. It will be degraded by gut digestive and liver enzymes. Increasing NAD levels using NAD precursors such as NMN can reverse the deleterious effects of NAD+ depletion. New studies have also shown that higher levels of NMN can increase stem cell regeneration and vascular health.

3 Main Pathways That Stimulate Anti-Aging

1. AMPK- a supplement
2. Sirtuin (NMN, NR, Resveratrol)
3. mTOR- (Rapamycin)

3 Stages Of Anti-Aging

Take Supplements-

1. Transcription Factors - read a gene and make a protein
2. Silencing Age Gene's-turn genes on and off quickly
3. Enzymes to turn on Sirtuins

Clip off acetyls spool up the DNA and silence aging

Deep Level of Aging

DNA Clock- tells typically what your genomic lifespan is measured by methylation reset or reverse with anti-aging compounds

2 Types of Enzymes:

Ones that add to methylation
Ones that subtract methylation

- Take enzymes that subtract methylation

3 Main Pathways That Regulate Aging

1. Serturins- Sirtuins are proteins that possess one of two types of enzymes:

1.) Mono-ADP-ribosyltransferase or
2.) Deacylase activity, including:

- deacetylase,
- desuccinylase,
- demalonylase,
- demyristoylase and
- depalmitoylase activity.

2. MTor- responds to how many amino acids you have in your body, Mtor hunkers down to protect your body the fewer amino acids it has access to
3. AMPK- energy sensor low levels of energy

Sirtuins

There are 7 sirtuin gene regulators (SIRT1–7). Sirtuins are thought to be responsible for the cardio-metabolic cause of the benefits of lean diets and exercise and when upregulated can delay key aspects of aging. However, nicotinamide adenine dinucleotide levels and sirtuin activity steadily decrease with age, but, Sirtuins benefit health in these ways as we age:

- SIRT1-

  - Protects against a decline in vascular function,
  - Protects against metabolic syndrome,
  - Protects against obesity
  - Protects against cardiomyopathy.

- SIRT3 is protective against risk that increase with age;

  - dyslipidemia
  - ischemia-
  - reperfusion injury

The decline of SIRT3 is further exacerbated by obesity and sedentary lifestyles. Activation of sirtuins or nicotinamide adenine dinucleotide repletion induces:

  - Angiogenesis,
  - insulin sensitivity,
  - Offers other health benefits
  - A factor in a wide range of age-related disorders
  - Improves cardiovascular and metabolic disease.

Sirtuin Therapy Future Outlook

Research continues to discover testing agents that activate SIRT1 and boost nicotinamide adenine dinucleotide levels. New discoveries are in progress all the time and many other substances show promise in their ability to improve the function of Sirtuins and the potential health improvements and longevity of humans is not only limited to cardiovascular and metabolic disease prevention and reversal in patients.

Epigenetics

The basis of age research is called epigenetics. By definition, this means the study of inherent changes in gene function. As we move through life, our genetic makeup changes in many different ways by many different causes. For instance, outside factors such as:

- Environmental Pollutants

  - Smog
  - Fires
  - Chemical Plants

- Smoking
- Alcohol
- Drug dependency
- High Stress
- Poor Stress Management
- Bad lifestyle habits

An unhealthy lifestyle, bad habits can bring about bad changes. And with a change in our genes, our bodies change as well. When the body changes, it starts to age. Whether these changes promote a predisposition to an inherited condition such as heart disease, diabetes or arthritis or create a new condition that the body remains unable to recover from, such epigenetic changes supply a lot of information for why these things happen. And when scientists find out why these changes happen they can work on a way of stopping them from happening, or even reversing them such as in aging.

The Best Anti-Aging Agent And Enzyme

Scientists have also determined an age reversing agent known as nicotinamide adenine dinucleotide or NAD+. This compound was present more in younger mice than older ones and is very important in repairing DNA damage. There is also another DNA repair enzyme called PARP1 Poly (ADP-ribose) polymerase 1 also known as NAD^+ ADP-ribosyltransferase 1 or poly (ADP-ribose) synthase 1 is an enzyme that in humans is encoded by the PARP1 gene. It is the most abundant of the PARP family of enzymes, accounting for 90% of the NAD+ used and which responds well to NAD+ levels in the human body. So the higher the NAD+ the more PARP1 enzyme your body will have.

Younger People Have Higher NAD+

Younger individuals have higher levels but levels start to fall as people age making it harder for DNA to restore itself with age. Scientists gave more NAD+ to older mice in research studies and found they started to appear younger, biologically, concluding that by changing adult cells into their earlier stage signs of age reversal is stimulated. It is important to take an NAD+ supplement and take better care of yourself to stop aging and damage at different levels. Once your cells are working well, they are in a better position to repair DNA and stop aging prematurely.

Genetic Health Component

Looking for a way to halt aging has undoubtedly stepped into science labs to unlock the mysteries of aging. In fact, research believes that not only may we be close to stopping aging but actually reversing it as well.

Your Genes Have A Big Role In How Fast Or Slow You Age

In the past, Genes were something beyond your control, but, now, here is what you need to know about genes and how they are affecting your aging process. DNA research has shown that specific genes are responsible for aging. Collectively dubbed as 'late life cyclers', this set of genes activate only in later life or during bouts of intense stress. Stressors related to aging such as molecular and cellular damage, oxidative stress and even some disease states cause these genes to respond.

Best Ways to Hack Your Genetics to Improve Your Health

- Lifestyle Factors That Affect Your Gene Health

    - Food and nutrition
    - You are what you eat. Your food choices can influence your future health.
    - Stress can activate your genes
    - Your moods can change your genetics.
    - If you stay in a stressed mood you will activate bad health genes
    - If you keep up happy hormones you activate good health genes
    - Everybody deals with stress, but too much, daily can activate genes for disease and have a negative impact on your health.
    - An active lifestyle will awaken the best genes.
    - Change your environment to one that supports good gene health.

Supplements To Help Prevent Some Types Of Cancer

- Organo-Germanium - GE-132
- Artemenisin
- Essiac Tea

- Vitamin C (Linus Pauling)
- DIM (reduces risk of some hormonal related types of cancer such as breast and prostate)

Age & Genetics

As we age it becomes harder for protein to get into the cells, the loss of protein metabolism can accelerate the onset of aging. Our genome can determine many aspects of our traits and health. Molecular processes allow our DNA (genotype) to affect our traits (phenotype). Your genotype is often connected to phenotype through protein expression and function which are involved in the formation of functional proteins. A person's genetic predisposition for an adult onset disease, such as high cholesterol or hypertension doesn't necessarily mean that person will develop those diseases, but their lifestyle habits will determine if and when the genes become activated. People who stay active, exercise, and who keep a healthy mindset and those who develop a daily routine of healthy lifestyle practices, tend to live longer. If you notice a rapid onset of aging see your doctor but also investigate your environment as exposure to certain toxins can activate genetic predisposition for disease. For example, mold allergies or illness can turn on the aging gene's and accelerate aging.

Anti-Aging Tips For More Youthful & Healthier DNA

- Stop Unhealthy habits
- Stay young at heart mindset
- Lower Stress Levels
- Exercise stay active daily
- Keep energy up be more active
- Take Anti-aging Supplements like NMN & Astragalus.
- Get Your Vitamin D levels up & daily dose of sunshine.
- Eat Omega 3's for a healthy heart and lubricate your system.
- Reverse the age clock with NMN & Resveratrol

Foods For Gene Health & Improved Stem Cell Production

Some of the best foods for stem cell growth are veggies that are full of the sulforaphane compound which boosts enzymes in the liver, to counteract harmful toxins we might digest or breathe in.

- **Cruciferous vegetables:**

- o Cauliflower,
- o Broccoli,
- o Kale,
- o Cabbage,
- o Bok choy,
- o Garden cress
- o Brussels sprouts

Foods For Healthy DNA

For healthier DNA, make the most of your diet by focusing on more nutrient-dense foods, such as:

- Colorful fruits
- Fresh vegetables,
- Whole grains,
- High-quality lean protein and
- Healthy fats.
- Eat Omega 3's for a healthy heart and lubricate your system

Even if you are healthy, to keep your DNA and Genes healthy, you will need to avoid:

- Processed foods

    - o Meats
    - o Dairy
    - o Junk foods
    - o Fast foods

- Highly refined foods
- Trans fats
- Refined sugars

Vitamin D Deficiency Related To Gene Expression

It sounds nearly impossible to be Vitamin D deficient, or for Vitamin D to affect your gene's but in fact, the *VDR* gene provides instructions for making a protein called vitamin D receptor (VDR), which allows the body to respond to vitamin D. Vitamin D deficiency is fairly common nowadays. Usually people are unaware that they are Vitamin D deficient until they begin to suffer with an associated health ailment. The first symptom often is you begin to feel unusually tired or depressed for no apparent reason, but Vitamin D deficiency causes many more serious problems than that.

How To Repair A Gene Error

Gene editing rewrites DNA, the biological code that makes up the instruction manuals of living organisms. With gene editing, researchers can disable target genes, correct harmful mutations, and change the activity of specific genes in plants and animals, including humans. Research has shown various genes can be repaired with amino acids and other various nutrients.

In genetic research, of just one of many vitamins; vitamin D supplementation improves the expression of 291 genes that are involved in apoptosis, immune function, transcriptional regulation, epigenetic modification, response to stress, cell cycle activity and differentiation. Unlike other vitamins, vitamin D functions like a hormone, and every single cell in your body has a receptor for it. The symptoms of Vitamin D deficiency are subtle or non-specific and without testing Vitamin D levels, there's no way to know if your symptoms are caused by low levels of vitamin D or some other health issue.

Symptoms Of Vitamin D Deficiency

Frequent colds, flu, respiratory tract infections like bronchitis and pneumonia additionally, vitamin D deficiency may cause the following:

- Chronic daytime fatigue
- Headaches
- Muscle aches
- Hair loss
- Bone pain
- Lower back pain
- Depressed mood
- Slow wound healing

If you have more than one of these symptoms, it's important to speak to your doctor and get a lab test.

Your body makes it from cholesterol when your skin is exposed to sunlight. It's also found in certain foods though it's very difficult to get enough from diet alone. Fortunately, vitamin D deficiency is usually easy to fix.

Foods & Lifestyle Habits To Increase Vitamin D:

- Increase your daily sunlight exposure to 20 Minutes
- Eat vitamin-D-rich foods such as:

  - Fatty fish (sardines, kipper, cod liver oil)
  - Dairy products.
  - Take a vitamin D supplement

Correcting a vitamin D deficiency is simple but it can offer many health benefits and great improvement of symptoms.

Genes Have An Effect On The Development Of Diseases

The ABO Gene

The ABO gene is a gene that is present in people with A, B, or AB blood types. The only blood type that doesn't have this gene is Type O. If you have the ABO gene and you live in an area with high pollution levels, you may be at a greater risk of heart problems than those who don't have the gene. The ABO gene can also increase your risk of coronary artery disease (CAD).

How To Lower Your ABO Risk

If you have the ABO gene, it doesn't automatically mean heart complications are going to be inevitable. There are ways to reduce and avoid further increasing your genetic risk of development. However, it is crucial to live in a clean environment and follow a heart healthy lifestyle:

- Stay away from highly polluted areas
- Home air filtration system
- Exercise regularly
- Exercise indoors if in a pollution zone.
- Maintain a heart-healthy diet

- Organic fruits, veggies, whole grains, fish, and nuts.
- Avoid smoking and other smokers
- Get regular physical exams
- Watch for warning signs
- Avoid GMO's (genetically modified)

ABO Gene Effect On Brain Health

The ABO gene is connected with brain function and memory loss. People who have blood types A, B, and AB are up to 82 percent more likely to develop cognition and memory problems which can lead to dementia compared to those with Type O. One possible reason for this memory loss is the fact that blood type can lead to things like high blood pressure, high cholesterol, and diabetes. These conditions can cause cognitive impairment and dementia.

Blood type has been connected with stroke, too, which can occur when the blood flow to the brain is disrupted.

Ways To Improve Brain Health:

- Avoid aluminum & heavy metal toxicity
- Eat Omega Rich Foods
- Exercise regularly.
- Do FIR detox sauna
- Avoid high stress.
- Sleep 7 to 9 hours nightly
- Drink water and occasionally distilled water

Cancer Effect On Genes & Aging

Cancer accelerates aging, some cancer treatments such as radiation therapy also ages the body 10+ years on average. Some genes have been studied to be more active in individuals with cancer, creating more responses in such people and signalling a higher level of distress. All of this activity will quickly age you taxing not only your looks but also your overall physical and mental health. The same set of genes are also activated if your circadian rhythm is out of sync.

The ABO gene may play a role with a heightened cancer risk, as well. This gene has been connected to other cancers, including lung, breast, colorectal, prostate, liver, and cervical cancers. This correlation has been studied for more than 60 years, and while research continues to show a correlation, there is no definitive explanation as to why the ABO gene may put you at a higher risk for some cancers.

What You Can Do if You're at Risk

While you may not be able to change your blood type, there are ways to lower your risk of cancer:

- Eat a healthy diet of fruits, vegetables, whole grains, fish, and poultry.
- Get regular exercise.
- Avoid smoking.

Though there are no sure ways to prevent cancer, these actions can help lower your risk and keep you healthy.

How Telomerase Reverse Aging

Everyday more compounds are researched in the search to find something that halts aging. The shortening of telomeres on the ends of DNA strands are associated with aging. The activity of the telomerase enzyme has been found to help slow the shortening but at present is still insufficient in completely restoring the lost telomeric DNA repeats and it doesn't completely stop cellular aging. However, counteracting the telomere shortening process is the enzyme, telomerase, that uniquely holds the key to delaying or even reversing the cellular aging process.

Healthy Genetics Due To Lifestyle Is A Factor In Longevity

A healthy lifestyle is one of the keys to longevity. For example, in Greece's there is the beautiful remote island, Ikaria, which has been named one of the healthiest places on earth because it is a hot spot for long living Greeks. In fact, there are more healthy people over 90 on the island of Ikaria than any other place on the planet.

Chapter 6

Longevity Zones
Around The Globe

Ikarian Longevity

The Ikarians of the Greek isles are active by second nature as it is a must by their landscape and demographic living situation. They get out and about daily and they exercise regularly as a part of their culture. The sunny Ikaria Island is located within a group of islands in the medeterainan sea within a "blue zone" where the people notoriously live long lives. What the typical "blue zone" research failed to recognize is the fact that all of the places listed in their "blue zones" include 3 other lifestyle factors that have been largely overlooked. Those two factors are:

1. They are located in relaxed communities
2. They have a special water quality source or they are in close proximity to glacial water or sea water. The blue zones are on either an island, a peninsula or in close proximity to the sea, ocean, glacial rivers or hot springs and the people bathe or use these natural water resources.
3. The people get out in nature daily, they work up a sweat and they have a little regular sun exposure.

Longevity Zone Diet Commonalities

Like the Medeterainian diet, Ikarians eat a variation of the typical food in the Mediterranean diet. Ikarians eat a diet consisting of natural unprocessed whole foods. Blue Zone diets are primarily plant-based, with as much as 95 percent of daily food intake coming from vegetables, fruits, grains, and legumes.

- Beans
- Lentils
- Chickpeas
- Black-eyed peas

A large part of their foods are beans and lentils which are an all natural, healthy and low-fat cholesterol-free source of protein and make a great meat substitute. They are a staple in Ikarian dishes and provide vitamins, minerals and antioxidants. They are also simple to cook, versatile, inexpensive and filling.

Longevity Zones

People in Longevity Zones typically avoid meat and dairy, as well as sugary foods and beverages. They stay physically active. For example, Ikarians dance daily and are literally running at 100 years old! There is science behind their long lives, it is the compounds in the foods that occur naturally in their healthy diet, the body chemicals they produce from truly living happily and additionally, their active lifestyle.

Ikaria Island Diet Staples Are:

- Wine (1-3 oz of their own preservative free blend)
- Fruits and
- Vegetables
- Whole grains
- Beans
- Potatoes
- Olive oil
- Eggs (1-3 per week)
- Meat (small portion fish, chicken & lamb weekly)
- Dairy (raw goat dairy products 1-3 per week)

The practice of eating and cooking with olive oil, which has cholesterol-lowering mono-unsaturated fats.

Ikaria Basic Breakfast Foods:

- Blue Zone Breakfast Basics:
- Cooked whole grains-
- Fruit & veggie smoothies
- Beans,
- Tofu scrambles

Ikaria Drinks

Blue zones rarely drink sodas and most centenarians drink:

- Water
- Tea
- Coffee
- Wine

Most centenarians in blue zones regions drink two to three cups of black coffee every day.

International Blue Zones

A blue zone is defined as a place where the environment is conducive to living to a ripe old age, in Ikaria residents are several times more likely to reach the age of 90 compared to other regions of the world.

1. Loma Linda, California USA
2. Okinawa, Japan
3. Costa Rica
4. Ikiria, Greece
5. Crete, Italy

Longevity Lifestyle Habits All Blue Zones Share

The whole of it is that longevity is attributed to the lifestyle of the blue areas. The lifestyle in each of these areas include the following daily lifestyle habits of the Blue Zone peoples that they all share in common amongst their populations:

- Living an active everyday lifestyle
- A calm mind practice effective stress management
- Avoidance of overindulgence or overeating
- Eat mostly plant-based diets
- Tea & Water consumption
- Participating in faith-based services
- Community and Family togetherness
- Staying socially active with other people and they express that they feel a sense of belonging and sense of purpose

Basically, the blue zones are communities of people who as a people they practice healthy lifestyle behaviors in a manner that the French describe as "Joie De Vivre".

The French Joie De Vivre

Joie de vivre is a French way of life, the phrase itself is often used by the English to express a cheerful enjoyment of life; an exultation of spirit. Joie De Vivre can be anything done with a sense of joy.

- joy of good conversation
- joy of shared togetherness
- joy of eating good things
- joy of having good drink
- joy of exploration
- joy of adventure
- joy of discovering new things
- joy of anything one might do.
- joy in facing the truths of life

Joie De Vivre

Joie de vivre may be seen as a joy of everything, a comprehensive joy, and living a lifetime with a philosophy that life is a joy. The next time you make a toast raise your glass to much joie de vivre!

- The quiet joy in being one's true self
- The savoring of the experience of life itself

No Happy, Healthy Person Wants To Die

Lifestyle Factors of Ikaria Greece

The topography of Ikaria makes physical activity a necessary part of the Ikarian lifestyle because of the terrain of the land, lack of transportation, hard work and a simple kind of life where all ages freely mingle within the culture as a whole. The young and the old share in the daily feast and joyous celebrations and festivities and enjoy daily after dinner parties, music and dancing. The kids play while the adults socialize and the elderly people are respected and loved by all those in their communities.

"Longevity Zones" Facts About World's Long Living People

- **Ikaria, Greece**- the island eight miles off the coast of Turkey in the Aegean Sea, they are isolated from the high stress world and have some of the world's lowest rates of middle-age diseases, mortality and dementia.
- **Okinawa, Japan**- Is an island off the coast of Japan in the China sea.
- **Crete Island**- Ogliastra Region, Sardinia Italy-
- **Loma Linda**- California USA the community is in southern California and it consists mostly of a faith based community that follows a lifestyle, spirituality, food, exercise, kindness and rest.
- **Nicoya Peninsula**- Costa Rica.

The Average Loma-Linda California Adventist, Lives 10 years Longer Than Average American Life Expectancy

Longevity Zones Beliefs & Sayings About Longevity

- **Ikaria, Greece** "We dominate time, time doesn't dominate us"
- **Okinawa, Japan** "We live out a happy life without regrets"

Longevity Zones People's Life Philosophy Phrases

- **Ikaria, Greece** "We Live Life To Live & To Feel" The Ikarians enjoy life and the simple daily pleasures in life give them great joy.
- **Okinawa, Japanese** - The Japanese phrase, "Nankurunaisa" which means "Everything will work out in the end" this is a reflection of how the Okinawan islanders think about their relaxed and optimistic attitude about life.

Longevity Zone Daily Activities

Ikarian Greeks- They do social activities and stay active in nature.

- Walking
- Swimming,
- Hiking,
- Dancing
- Socializing.
- Emotionally Supportive

- Story telling
- Laughter & Talking
- Joyful Spirit
- All-Is-One "We" mindset
- Loving hearted people

The blue zones typically have a culture that is emotionally supportive of each other so that no one feels left out or isolated from birth into old age resulting in low rates of mental illness.

Shangrila Long Lifer's

The infamous Shangri La, is believed to have been in the Hunza Valley region of northern Pakistan. Hunza is in an isolated area of the Himalayas. The Hunzas are a long-living people said to live up to 145 years old but not scientifically documented. The Hunza people are not plagued with the typical adult onset diseases and have a very low incidence of cancer. They do in fact live long healthy lives but it's impossible to determine just how old they are because in their culture they do not keep up with birthdays so no one can really determine their true ages which is one reason they are not included in the list of blue zones.

Hunza Geography

Hunza is a very remote place 100 miles long and 2 miles wide sitting at an elevation of 8500 feet situated in the western part of the Himalayan mountains. Hunza is home to a community of people said to survive longer than any society on Earth. Some say Hunza native people live to be 150 years old which is unproven, thus far, due to poor record keeping. Regardless, they do live very long lives. The lifestyle habits of these people are:

- Grow their own food and do not have junk food
- Drink fresh glacier water that is white in color from high mineral and calcium content.
- Bath in glacier water springs.
- Happy mindset
- Deal swiftly with stress
- Stay active
- Work hard
- They only eat 3 oz of meat per month or less.

In Hunza people claim they live long lives because of their gene's and claim they are the descendants of Alexander the Great. The people are hard workers, they work cultivating, growing, harvesting and consuming fresh foods.

Hunza Region Food Staples

- Apricots
- Apricot Kernels
- Apricot Oil
- Wheat
- Breads (variety of types)
- Wheat-based dishes
- Buckwheat
- Barley
- Millet
- Rice
- Corn
- Rye

Fruits

- Apricots
- Mulberries
- Grapes
- Oranges
- Apples
- Pears
- Peaches
- Cherries
- Mellons
- Tomatoes

Vegetables:

- Leafy greens
- Potatoes
- Carrots
- Squash
- Turnips
- Onions

- Garlic
- Cabbage
- Sprouts

Protein:

- Dried beans
- Peas
- Nuts
- Seeds

The Hun's Unique Eating Habits

The Hunza people grow apricot trees abundantly everywhere. Apricots are an important staple in the Hunza diet. They eat:

- fresh apricots,
- dried apricots,
- apricot soup,
- mashed apricot sauces, (with a variety of spices)
- apricot preserves,
- apricot juice,
- apricot bread,
- apricot cake,
- apricot pie and they drink
- apricot infused glacier water

The Hunzas even blend apricots together with apricot kernel milk and mix it with snow to make apricot ice cream. The Hunza diet consisted of raw milk, not pasteurized, they rarely eat meat but they occasionally cook with bone broth, fresh grains and veggies. They eat very little sugar and as nomads and herders, they naturally get plenty of exercise. The other characteristic that is unique about the Hunzas is that they eat massive amounts of apricot products and they even eat the apricot seed kernels.

Longevity Power Of Apricots

Apricots are one of the best foods next to turmeric for tumour eradication as apricot kernels contain the glycoside compound, amygdalin. Laetrile is a compound of amygdalin that can potentially help heal various cancers, including breast cancer. Laetrile is sourced from apricot kernels, amygdalin is also vitamin B17. Unfortunately, if you eat too much it can be a danger to health, as well, but the truth is that apricot kernels have been consumed in small quantities for their nutritional and healing properties for thousands of years, especially by people in the cool, arid areas where apricot trees are indiginous and they grow, naturally without cultivation.

Lifestyle Rules Of Hunza People:

- Eat a diet of fresh fruits and vegetables
- Fasting one day a week
- Daily Physical Exercise
- Live Frugally, they aren't wasteful
- Conqueror's spirit of life

Proud Heritage

Lastly, the Hunza people claim to be the proud descendants of Alexander the Great; they claim their ancestors settled there when remnants of his troops settled in this remote Himalayan village around 350 BC.

Habits Of The Oldest People In Japan

Some of the oldest living people documented have been Japanese. In particular, the Okinawan Islanders, that have a special lifestyle and way of life.

- The people are gentle, laid back, they enjoy nature in its splendor.
- Many people vacation on Okinawa island to enjoy the natural hot spring baths to relax and rejuvenate.
- The Okinawan diet is filled with soy-based foods such as tofu and miso soup.
- Their traditional daily diet is several servings of vegetables and soy plus a serving of fruit, daily.
- Sweet potatoes are eaten often as well as other vegetables which are eaten with the peel on.

Other common vegetables that are eaten daily are rice, bitter gourds, chives, radish, onions, cabbages, bok choy, carrots and leafy greens and all of these foods have anti-aging, anti-inflammatory and blood purifying properties. There are many types of Miso but the original was brought from China, via the Korean Peninsula, made of a fermented spice, ground fish, meat and salt, and a type of fermented soybeans or millet.

- Okinawans eat miso, broth and stock soups on a regular basis and even eat soups for breakfast.
- Tofu is traditional in Japan, but Okinawan jimami tofu is made from peanuts and potato starch.
- They eat condiments daily. They eat black sugar syrup as a dessert,
- They eat fermented condiments such as soy sauce and miso.
- They eat raw garnishes, a dab of wasabi and grated ginger.
- They eat small servings of caviar or fish eggs, fish and seafood.
- They eat Umi budo, a grape like sea vegetable, is used as a garnish for sushi and many other types of food or it is often eaten plain or with soy sauce or vinegar.

Okinawans use seaweed as a base flavoring in their soups and often make soups with bone broths which are high in collagen, minerals and thyroid boosters for good metabolism, healthy hair skin and nails which provide them with youthful skin and lasting beauty.

Miso is a staple in the Japanese diet, it is made of fermented soup base. It is a food made of aged, fermented rice, barley, and soybeans. It is a staple of the Asian diet, too. Miso paste was a way the ancients preserved food that originated in China and was later introduced by buddhist pricsts to the Japanese over 1,300 years ago. It was made with fermented mixtures of salt, grains, and soybeans.

In Asia, Miso and Rice are like Meat and Potatoes in the Americas'.

Health research studies indicate that eating miso can help:

- Reduced risks of various cancers:

  - Breast
  - Uterine
  - Lung
  - Prostate
  - Colon cancer
  - Radiation protection

Miso Soup Recipe

2 Cups Water (boiling)
2 T Soy Sauce (optional)
1 T Miso
¼ Cup of sea kelp or sea veggies
1 T chives (as topper garnish)
Optional: fish, rice or soy curls

Life Details About The Oldest Living Man

- **Jiroemon Miyake Kimura - Age 116 from Okinawa**

  o Jiroemon was health-conscious and active.
  o Born in the fishing village of Kamiukawa, Japan
  o He lived in Kyōtango, Kyoto, "Kyoto by the sea".
  o Jiroemon woke up early each morning
  o He read the daily newspaper.
  o He finished school second in his class.
  o He worked in a post office for 45 years.
  o He was sociable & enjoyed talking to people.
  o After retiring he farmed until the age of 90
  o He credited his longevity to his diet and only eating small portions of food.
  o In Okinawa it is said at dinner, "hara hachi bu" which means "eat until you are 80% full".
  o He was a father of several children.
  o All of his siblings lived long lives, 90-110.
  o He farmed as a pastime after retirement.
  o He ate a breakfast of rice porridge and miso soup
  o He drank ginseng, turmeric tea and Agari tea after a meal, Agaria is a powdered tea created from the dust, buds and small leaves left over from the processing of fine green teas.
  o He dined on tofu, rice, bamboo shoots, seaweed, ginger, pickles, fish, nori, sushi and a little bit of cake.
  o He enjoyed Dashi, a stock made from kelp and bonito fish flakes, which serves as the base for most Okinawan soups
  o He ate natural foods native to Japan and followed wellness rituals related to his culture. Tofu skin, yuba, bean curd skin, bean curd sheet, or bean curd robes, is a food product made from soybeans.
  o He partook in his community fish market events, visiting which is famous for fresh seafood, red Kasumi crab and sushi.

"For Centuries, the Chinese Revere the Okinawa Island as the Land of the Immortals."

Unique Environmental Factors In Kyoto Beach Japan

The sand on Kyoto beach is 75 % quartz, and when rubbed it vibrates and sounds like music some say waking in the sand balances the body's vibrational frequencies for better health.

- Many Japanese people go on holiday in Kyoto to breathe in the invigorating sea air, soak in the revitalising hot springs and enjoy the seafood, crabs, sushi and the rare sea vegetable. Umi budo referred to as *"Green Caviar"* is a delicacy sea plant that only grows in the northern-most area of Okinawa Island it is one of the only places on the planet where the plant is able to survive.

Typically, the only meat Okinawans typically eat is seafood, they generally do not eat other types of meat as it's kind of hard to keep livestock on an island and those Okinaawans that do eat meat, eat very little, in fact, most Okinawans do not eat any other type of meat and only a low percentage of their diet are eggs and dairy. This means their diet on average, is approximately 95 percent plant-based with mostly sea vegetables and other vegetables, rice and other typical regional foods. The Okinawa diet limits several types of foods such as, fruit, meat, dairy, nuts, seeds and processed carbs.

We have reviewed what many of the oldest living people ate in their diets and we've considered their habits and lifestyle factors as well. Now, it is time to take a look into our own diet and the ways of cleaning it up to activate our inner fountain of youth.

Chapter 7

Anti-Aging Foods
As Medicine

Hipocrates Was Right About Health & Longevity

Turns out the father of modern medicine was right all along. In the emerging fields of nutrigenomics and nutrigenetics scientific research has now proven that what Hipocraties said all those many years ago about our food being our medicine, was correct.

"Let thy food be thy medicine and thy medicine be thy food" Hipocrates

Dr. Hippocrates prescribed lifestyle modifications such as diet and exercise to treat diseases. The role of nutrition in the health and wellbeing of the human body is of the utmost importance and in fact, the foods we eat determines our future health prognosis and longevity outcome. Today, we know that various diseases, including cardiovascular disorders, metabolic syndrome, neurological diseases, and type 2 diabetes have roots in our genetics that are in-turn influenced by our diet, nutritional choices, and lifestyle factors. For example, the intake of a diet rich in niacin, magnesium and folate have proved to be beneficial in providing protective effects against the development of lung cancer in Hispanic population of smokers, who have a higher susceptibility of suffering from this disease. Incorporating these protective nutrients showed an enhanced DNA repair capacity toward double-strand DNA breaks, a mechanistic biomarker strongly linked to acquisition of lung cancer gene methylation in smokers. Optimal intakes of the nutrients above was found to reduce the methylation by up to 36%.

Food Intake and Its Impact on Evolution

The important factor in gene activation is environmental factors which include the effects on genes regarding the foods we eat. Our diet impacts our genome and metabolism over a long period of time and influences genetic changes in future generations of our offspring.

Food Intolerances & Allergies

Various food intolerances affect various ethnic groups across the globe and have developed over time due to the diets of our ancestors. Today, the chemicals used in food processing and preservation pose a toxic risk factor to good health. Humans were hunter gatherers, and it is difficult for the body to metabolise artificial chemicals which often biological transmutations in the body into a substance the body can recognise and metabolise, such as estradiol, a bad cancer causing estrogen and endocrine disruptor thereafter creating mass chaos in the metabolic system turning our inner fountain of youth into a muddy stagnant cesspool. That is why it is important to keep your diet wholesome.

"The Downfall Of Man's Health Began With The First Processed Food, Bread." Summer Perry

Since then, it has been found that the people of Finland and northern European cultures are exceptionally lactose tolerant people while a large population of Asia are lactose intolerant and do not digest milk and dairy products very well. A study suggests that around 86% of Chinese study groups are lactose intolerant. In the U.S. many people are gluten intolerant and have food allergies. The most common food allergies are:

- Shellfish
- Peanuts,
- Eggs,
- Dairy and
- Wheat.

It is thought that mold may play a role in the high occurrence of these types of allergies due to a person's allergic reaction to the mold mycotoxins in these types of foods. If you find yourself sneezing a lot around meal times it is recommended to have food allergy testing.

The Worst Processed Foods Of All: White Sugar And Flour

What do you get when you mix water in with a bowl of sugar? Syrup. What happens if you mix water in with a bowl of white flour? You get glue paste. White sugar and flour turns your inner fountain of youth into a syrupy sticky stagnant mess that eventually acts as glue blocking the flow of your inner fountain of youth. White sugar is one of the most highly toxic processed food toxins on the planet. First of all, any food that is white is highly bleached with carcinogens. High sugar intake in a simple carbohydrate and starchy carb diets lead to an increased risk of heart disease. Excessive simple sugars lead to a high insulin state which, in turn, is the primary trigger of high triglycerides, a type of blood fat, and very low-density lipoproteins (VLDL). We will look at the mechanism of action in more detail later. Suffice to say that both triglyceride and VLDL are independent risk factors for atherosclerosis. In addition, sugar lowers good HDL cholesterol, raises bad LDL cholesterol, resulting in a rise in total cholesterol. It is estimated that a high sugar intake may account for as many as 150,000 premature deaths from heart disease in the US each year.

Cleopatra's Diet

Cleopatra is one of the world's most renowned beauties. She was a strikingly beautiful woman and cultivated some of the world's first beauty practices. Cleopatra had a beautiful face and body. Therefore, one would find interest in what she ate in her daily diet which consisted of the following.

- Fruit- Figs, Dates, Peaches, Pomegranates
- Nuts- filberts, walnuts, pine kernels, pistachios
- Extra-virgin olive oil,
- Goat milk cheeses,
- Honey
- Wine
- Vegetables, (artichokes, olives, radishes)
- Legumes and lentlls
- Grains, (tiny grains, cous-cous)
- Aromatic herbs (rosemary, parsley, mint, sage and cinnamon)
- Wild Boar & Birds
- Fish,
- Lotus
- Water from the Nile "The Giver Of Life"

Anti Aging Super Foods From The Sea

Roe and Caviar are sources of vitamins and minerals, including anti-aging super omega 3 fatty acids, which helps to promote healthy skin, hair, nails as well as support a healthy nervous system, circulatory system and immune system.

- Caviar are fish eggs from sturgeon
- Tobiko are fish eggs from flying fish
- Ikura are fish eggs from salmon
- All caviar are referred to as "fish-roe."

Why You Should Eat Caviar

Caviar is an anti-aging super food. One one ounce serving of caviar has an adult's daily requirement of Vitamin B12 in its natural form without the dangers of synthetic B12. Caviar contains Omega 3 fatty acids, Omegas are essential fats that must be consumed in your diet because your body does not produce them. Other nutrients found in Caviar include vitamins A, B6, E, Iron, Magnesium, DHA, EPA's and Selenium. All anti-aging brain food.

- True Beluga caviar is the roe from only one type of fish, the beluga sturgeon which originated in the triassic period and it is a living prehistoric fish.
- Beluga caviar is currently illegal in the U.S.A.
- The Fish and Wildlife Service banned the import of all Beluga products from the Caspian Sea.
- Eggs are filled with Omegas.
- One one ounce serving of fish eggs contains

  o 420 milligrams of the omega-3 fatty acid EPA
  o 600 milligrams of DHA.

Roe Is A Nutritional Super Food

Roe is the perfect addition to most diet:

- Paleo
- Keto

Roe is:

- Carb-free,

- Sugar-free,
- Low glycemic index

Roe is:

  o (64%) fat
  o High quality essential nutrients:

    ▪ B vitamins
    ▪ Choline
    ▪ Magnesium
    ▪ Selenium
    ▪ Vitamin K2
    ▪ Calcium
    ▪ Vitamin A
    ▪ Zinc
    ▪ Iodine
    ▪ DHA
    ▪ Vitamin D
    ▪ Trace minerals

Eat Truffles For Anti-Aging

Truffles grow underground and are similar to a mushroom and are a great source of antioxidants, compounds that help fight free radicals and prevent oxidative damage to your cells. Studies show that antioxidants are important to many aspects of your health and may even be linked to a lower risk of chronic conditions, such as cancer, heart disease and diabetes

Truffles For Hormones

Truffles contain Androstenone, a hormone chemical that mimics our reproductive pheromones that is also the molecule of the smell of truffles. Some describe the scent as being a musky aroma. Apparently, it is a similar smell of the hormones of a male boar because it has been claimed that it actually makes female pigs go into mating stance. Androstenone is a steroidal pheromone. A form of it is found in boar's saliva. It is also found in celery cytoplasm. Androstenone was the first mammalian pheromone to be identified. Truffles are arousing and slightly intoxicating, in a way.

Truffles For Great Skin

Truffles are great for your skin because they contain essential fatty acids such as omegas. When used in beauty products they help to diminish the look of wrinkles. They provide super hydration to skin and hair as well. The scent of truffles is used in fragrances as a pheromone attractant. Truffles are a sign of luxury and extravagance.

Studies testing a very strong truffle extract showed that truffles may:

- Lower stress
- Lower cortisol
- Lower blood pressure
- Lower cholesterol.
- Control blood sugar.
- Protect your liver from damage.
- Reduce inflammation
- Fight bacterial infections.
- Help prevent cancer.

Mushrooms Mycoceutics

Mushrooms are a superfood, with the immune boosting powers of beta glucans. There are a family of mushrooms with life saving benefits. Some of the most known mushrooms for longevity and anti-aging benefits also boost the lymphatic system and lymph fluid functions are:

- Chaga
- Mitake
- Reshi
- Turkey Tail
- Lions Mane
- Shiitake

Shiitake mushrooms are high in protein and make a great meat replacement. If you're trying to cut back on red meat but still love a burger, the cap of one shitake mushroom is about the size of a quarter-pound burger and if you season it just right, you'll never miss the meat. They are great as a topper for almost all dishes. Caution must be used when harvesting mushrooms as some are poisonous it is best to purchase from an experienced supplier.

Quality Of Foods

Sometimes longevity is not only about the quality of food we eat, it is also about fasting. Fasting triggers Autophagy, the body's internal self cleaning mechanisms. Fasting can be easy if you support your body with drinks that stimulate the autophagy processes in the body.

Food & Intermittent Fasting

Breakfast- (breaking overnight fast/1st food of day)

- The first food you put in your stomach regulates gut bacteria and hunger hormone release for the rest of the day, therefore breakfast is the most important meal of the day.
- View breakfast as breaking athopahgy, while in a fast, hunger is your friend triggering the self-eating mechanisms to clean up protein waste and do its inner self-cleaning.
- You can eat your 1st meal of the day at various times. Drink warm and cold fluids and water as long as you can before breaking your fast, but do not drink anything 30 minutes prior to eating to allow gastric juices to accumulate in the stomach for digestion.
- If you experience detox nausea, break your fast with grapefruit slices or another favorite citrus or green leafy salads or steamed spinach, this will help alleviate the nausea instantly and balance the digestion and hunger hormones.
- Along with your first foods include a teaspoon of kimchi or a fermented food, such as coconut yogurt, that contains good bacteria.
- For people sensitive to dairy here are some excellent dairy-free ways to work plenty of enzymes and probiotics into your diet. Foods that curb your hunger hormones and support your gut bacteria are:

  - Coconut Yogurt/Kefir
  - Kombucha Tea
  - Tempeh
  - Kimchi
  - Sauerkraut
  - Pickles/Pickled Okra/ Pickled Beets
  - Pickled fruits and vegetables
  - Cultured condiments/Coconut aminos
  - Dandelion
  - Onion
  - Jicama

Additionally, supplement your diet with foods containing prebiotics and probiotics.

Autophagy For Anti-Aging Eating Pattern
Breakfast- Water, tea's, coffee
Lunch- Smoothie (with anti-aging add ons)
Dinner-Balanced Diet (1 item from each food group)
Snacks- Plant-based- Vegetable or Whole Fruit (3 x day)
Fasting- 7pm until late breakfast

Nutrition for Sex

Humans are made to enjoy love and intimacy for a lifetime. Nitric Oxide (NO) is the nutrient that puts the "O" in "DynOmite" and "Orgasm" that's why foods that contain NO are known as they are aphrodisiac foods. Some of these supercharged sex-aid foods are:

Foods Packed With Nitric Oxide:

- Arugula
- Rhubarb
- Kale
- Swiss
- Chard
- Spinach
- Bok Choy
- Beets

Foods Packed With Antioxidants

- Berries
- Grapes
- Pomegranates
- Apples
- Figs

Super Antioxidants

Proanthocyanidins are a group of phyto-nutrients that are 50 times more powerful than vitamin E and 30 times more potent than vitamin C, as an antioxidant. Proanthocyanidins include:

- Red grapes.
- Black grapes.
- Grape seeds.
- Red wine.
- Bilberries.
- Cranberries.
- Strawberries.
- Blueberries.

Anthocyanins

Another super antioxidant is thirty times more potent than vitamin C in comparison to the elimination of free radical damage are anthocyanins, for example, purple cabbage contains more than 36 types of anthocyanins, making it an excellent source of anthocyanins. Purple cabbage is a rich source of anthocyanins, which are beneficial plant compounds that may reduce your risk of all forms of heart disease.

Drinks Filled With Antioxidants

- Green Tea
- Oat Milk
- Cranberry Juice
- Pineapple Juice
- Celery Juice

Chapter 8
Youthful Hair, Skin & Nails

Signs Of Aging

Some of the most visible signs of the aging process can be seen in our skin, hair and nails. There are many ways to combat the signs of aging and to activate the inner fountain of youth within your hair, skin and nails.

Skin:

Your skin can absorb what you use on it so it's important to use clean natural products without a lot of artificial chemicals. The best way to activate your skin's inner fountain of youth is to supplement it with skin nutrition, anti-aging therapies and skincare. For example:

- **Collagen Supplement** -ingestible bone broth or multi-collagen powder added to a drink or smoothie.
- **Dry Brush Skin**- Use a dry brush to get your lymph flowing, the lymphatic system is a part of your inner fountain of youth, dry brushing is an activator, brush toward heart, head to toe and back up toward your heart.
- **Detox Baths**- take baths daily use epsom salts, baking soda, magnesium bath and do heavy metal detox baths.
- **Clean Personal Care Products**- many body products expose you to hundreds of chemicals daily.
- **Reduce negative thoughts and interactions**- negative emotions produce damaging chemicals and hormones that turn on fight or flight mechanisms and stress the body, accelerating aging.
- **Use Moisturizers**- Hyuralonic acid and 100% natural face oil blends
- **Activate Autophagy**- self-eating of internal dead cells and renewal of internal and external skin cells
- **Bedtime regime**- always take off your makeup with good quality cleanser, water, spring water, evian water or oil cleansers and then hydrate with a night serum and face cream, we recommend anti-aging brand wrinkle cream and face lift serum.

- **Water filtration system**- clean chemical-free water and occasional distilled water. Avoid dead water.
- **Lymphatic drainage**- is a massage technique that helps you to prevent lymph stagnation, your lymph is part of your inner fountain of youth so keep it flowing.
- **Facial massages** - rose oil, frankincense, buchinol vibration circulation tightening energizing aromatherapy
- **Exfoliation**-off with the old dead cells and energise the new, use a fruit enzyme like alpha hydroxy acids, or try a coffee scrub, exfoliation on extremities to reduce the appearance of cellulite.
- **Caffeine topical** and drinking it in tea
- **Diet**- take a multi and fill up on plants, fruits and veggies. Make sure you get the RDA of essential nutrients, especially those that affect our inner fountain of youth, such as Vitamin D- absorbed by sunlight and D3 gives us energy, radiance and strong teeth and bones to prevent bone loss as we age.
- **Blockers Of Intercellular Communications**- rid your body of the blockers of cell communications, they act as beaver-dam and block the flow of our inner fountain of youth, making it stagnant. These hidden culprits are pathogens such as yeast or mold which congest our liver and lymph nodes and are also dna blockers.
- **Mindset**- be open minded, keep in touch with your youth. Live in a state of peace and harmony. Stress hormones accelerate aging. Stressing eventually shows signs in your appearance.
- **Empty Feelings**- fill up happiness instead of food. try new things so you never feel bored. Watch comedy and get the feel-good, happy hormones flowing in your inner fountain of youth.
- **External products** - you do not want to put anything on your skin that once absorbed may block the pores and elimination processes of your skin, which is an excretory organ so use clean products that are all natural and chemical-free and detoxifying.
- **Exercise**- Invigorate your body by staying active, helps collagen production and skin tightening, it also helps your inner fountain of youth produce many feel good hormones that put a smile on your face, too, many good things are produced during exercise including detoxification through sweat and burning off stored fat.
- **Weight Management**- staying at a healthy weight is great for anti-aging as it reduces your risk of stretched out skin and obesity related diseases. Additionally, your heart has to pump through an additional mile of blood vessels for every extra pound of fat stored on your body which is exhausting to your inner fountain of youth.

Excess Stored Fat=Toxins

Ceramides An Oily Fountain Of Youth

Fats are important but there are good and bad ones. Ceramides are the best fats for anti-aging in your skin and hair. Ceramides are a class of fatty acids called lipids. They're naturally found in skin cells and make up about 50% of your outer layer of skin, the epidermis. Ceramides are lipids that help form the skin's barrier and ceramides help your skin retain moisture.

Ceramides also help your skin protect against environmental aggressors like toxins and pollution. Without the proper ratio of ceramides, the skin's barrier can become compromised, leading to breakouts, dryness, wrinkles, itching, rashes, irritation and that's why it's important to include foods that contain ceramides in your diet.

Foods that are good sources of ceramides are:

- Soy beans,
- Sweet potatoes
- Eggs,
- Brown rice
- Dairy,
- Wheat germ

Caution: Refrain from using oral ceramide supplements as they can negatively alter your lipid profile.

We Need Vitamin D, Without Sun Damage

Rapid Skin Aging May Be Caused By Deficiencies

One example is a vitamin D deficiency. Low vitamin D levels has a negative effect on more than just your bones, it affects your skin health, too. Healthy vitamin D levels help to prevent premature skin aging. Still important to protect your skin from the sun because too much sun leads to accelerated skin aging, also.

Sun Produces Vitamin D But Causes Sun Damage

It's almost an oxymoron and it is a paradoxical health delima that humans need sunshine to stay healthy but at the same time the sun causes sun damage and free radical damage. There is a happy medium and part of it has to do with the chemicals we consume and the reaction our biofilm and sweat content has on the surface layers of our skin when it comes in contact with the sun. Just as in lab animals during scientific cancer research studies, scientists use to give the mice burned processed meat to induce cancer then study various substances to cure the mice. If we eat a lot of processed junk and then burn our skin in the sun over time it may have a similar effect. Even if we eat all organic, we still have to protect our skin as UVA and UVB rays are present outside in sunlight and even in the shade. Direct exposure cooks our skin in a way, stimulating melanin in defense, thus the reason we tan. Plants make their own concoction of chemicals to stay safe in the sun, too and in the right environment, in a more effective way than humans. The sun is good for us, just as it is for the plants, as it helps us produce vitamin D.

Vitamin D3 The Anti-Wrinkle Vitamin/Hormone

Vitamin D3 reduces the progerin production that causes wrinkles and alleviates most Hutchinson-Gilford progeria syndrome (HGPS) features, an extremely rare genetic disorder that causes premature, rapid aging shortly after birth. It has been discovered that de novo point mutations in the LMNA gene have been found in individuals with HGPS, too. D3 also slows down epigenetic aging in overweight and obese non-HGPS individuals with suboptimal vitamin D status. The sun gives us Vitamin D that our bodies use to help our skin and bones stay strong. Sunscreen was invented to keep you safe from the sun's rays while outside.

Skin Aging & Oxidative Stress

Exposure to ultraviolet (UV) radiation ages the skin more quickly. The skin is one of the largest organs in the body. Skin aging in older adults is manifested by increased numbers of pigmented spots, wrinkles and features of sagging. Because the skin derives much of its oxygen from the atmosphere it also derives free radical oxygen species in the same way and this increases oxidative stress. Other environmental exposures, especially to cigarette smoking and UV light, also predispose to oxidative stress by both increasing free radical oxygen species and reducing the activity of antioxidant enzymes. In addition to these changes, the skin becomes more predisposed to neoplastic changes with age; again, increased oxidative stress may contribute to this. There is some evidence that UV light also impairs the immune function of the skin through altering antioxidant enzyme levels that impact on the number of Langerhans cells in the epidermis. There are a lot of government regulations for sunscreen activities and in some counties, such as Australia, it is against the law to send your children outdoors without hats for sun protection. Using a daily sunscreen is essential, there are thousands of chemical sunscreen options or if you greatly limit your sun exposure you may consider trying an essential plant oil that offers natural sun protection and it is always imperative to protect your skin's inner fountain of youth.

Sunscreen

There are two general types of sunscreens, chemical and physical.

- A chemical sunscreen absorbs the UV rays.
- physical sunscreen reflects the harmful rays away from the skin like a temporary coat of armor.

Sunblock

There are two types of physical sunblocks that are mostly used:

- Zinc oxide and
- Titanium dioxide.

Both provide broad-spectrum UVA and UVB protection. They are gentle enough for everyday use, especially for individuals with sensitive skin and for children, because they rarely cause skin irritation. But, because of scattering effect, they often causes so

Sun Filters

- Plant oils
- Hats &
- Protective clothing

Plants do not typically sunburn because of their essential oils and phytonutrients that offer sun protection and many of these plant extracts offer us sun protection qualities, too.

Plants

Produce their own chemical sunscreens that protect them from harmful ultraviolet light. These chemical sunscreens protect plants from harmful solar radiation while still allowing them to carry out photosynthesis, which is driven by sunlight. The plant's sun block is actually a combination of special molecules that form in the plant's tissue. These molecules join together to create a compound that blocks the ultraviolet light. But at the same time, these compounds still allow other kinds of sunlight to pass through. That way, the plant can still make its own food without withering or cooking in sunlight.

Herbal Sunscreen

Herbs and herbal preparations have a high potential due to their antioxidant activity, primarily. Antioxidants such as vitamins (vitamin C, vitamin E), flavonoids, and phenolic acids play the main role in fighting against free radical species that are the main cause of numerous negative skin changes. Although isolated plant compounds have a high potential in protection of the skin, whole herbs extracts showed better potential due to their complex composition. Many studies showed that green and black tea (polyphenols) ameliorate adverse skin reactions following UV exposure. The gel from aloe is believed to stimulate skin and assist in new cell growth. Spectrophotometer testing indicates that as a concentrated extract of Krameria triandra it absorbs 25 to 30% of the amount of UV radiation typically absorbed by octyl methoxycinnamate. Sesame oil resists 30% of UV rays, while coconut, peanut, olive, and cottonseed oils block out about 20%. A "sclerojuglonic" compound which is forming from naphthoquinone and keratin is the reaction product that provides UV protection.

Traditional Natural Plant Sunscreens

- Keratin
- Sclerojuglonic
- Naphthoquinone
- Krameria triandra

Sunshine, Nature and Fresh Air Are
Daily Essentials For Longevity

Sunshine And Heat Autophagy

Although it is important for anti-aging to protect your skin from the sun by wearing sunscreen. Sunshine and fresh air are an essential part of a healthy lifestyle. In addition to the benefit of sunshine in the body by making vitamin D, additionally, new research proves that the heat from the sun has health benefits, too. Mild heat stress for one hour can stimulate autophagy and initiate the body's self-cleaning mode known as autophagy, that helps the body clean itself internally to get rid of dead and dying cells while stimulating renewal cell growth. If you prefer to stay out of the sun, you can utilize alternative heat therapies to stimulate autophagy such as:

- Hot water immersion
- Steam sauna or Hot sauna
- Localized heat applications

    o Hot stone massage
    o Hot mud mask

Heat therapies may provide many therapeutic benefits, particularly in conditions with dysfunctional autophagy. 120 degrees fahrenheit is the maximum safe hot water temperature that should be delivered from a fixture. Therefore, do not allow hot water above 100 degrees fahrenheit to touch your skin as it can be considered hazardous. For more information about skincare and the simple way to keep your skin looking youthful for life, read my other book "Beyond Beautiful Skin". It's loaded with skin care tips including a home face-lift technique.

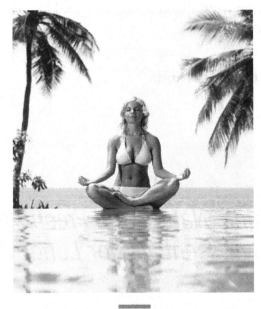

Hair Growth

Bergamot oil may help to promote hair growth. One study found that bergamot essential oil helps facilitate wound healing and reduce inflammation. This may help promote hair growth and a healthy scalp. Another study found that bergamot displays antimicrobial activity when applied to the scalp.

Hair Thinning & Loss Prevention

There are several natural substances that can help prevent age related hair loss. For example, Redensyl is an extract from the Larch tree and Green Tea. Proven to increase the number of growing hairs while reducing the number of dying hairs in under 60 days.

- Use a hair growth serum.
- Try that is one of the most effective ways to regrow hair quickly but there are other plant extracts that also help hair growth.
- Capixyl, proven to increase hair shaft thickness and health
- Biotin vitamin B is one of the most common hair loss vitamins
- Keratin protein is a common hair health treatment

Faster Hair Growth With L-Cysteine

L-Cysteine is a hair growth amino acid that helps hair grow 300% faster and it is the main component of Keratin protein.
Some L-Cysteine rich foods are:

- sage
- meat,
- dairy products,
- eggs,
- nuts,
- seeds, and
- legumes.

L-Cysteine is also abundant in protein powders used in weight-loss and body-building shakes and smoothies.

Simple Ways to Make Your Hair Grow Faster
- Get frequent trims to eliminate brittle ends

- Resist the urge to chemically treat
- Avoid overprocessing with hair dye, perms & relaxers
- Minimize heat use
- Use ion ceramic hair styling tools to reduce damage
- Brush daily to distribute your hair's natural oils to ends
- Eat the right hair nourishing Vitamin B & protein rich foods
- Skip a day or two between shampooing
- Use a deep conditioning repair mask
- Take a daily mult-ivitamin, multi-mineral, multi-amino acid
- Finish your shower with a cool rinse to seal the cuticle.

Aging Hair And How To Restore It

A tell tale sign of aging is dull, lackluster, thinning hair and a receding hairline. Keratin is the protein that is essential for healthy hair and as we age it is harder for the body to utilize and absorb vital essential fatty acids and nutrients. Additionally, hormonal declines or imbalances associated with aging show in the health of your hair.

Ceramides make the hair shiny and lustrous looking. Ceramides are kind of like an oily glue that holds your hair's cuticles together. There are three types of oils found in the hair cuticle:

1. Ceramide
2. Cholesterol
3. Methyl Eicosanoic Acid (MEA)

Ceramides Are The Fountain Of Youth For Your Hair

There are many benefits of Ceramides for your hair. For every strand of hair to be strong, keep its elasticity, retain moisture and porosity, keep its shine and smoothness, and be resistant to breakages and weathering, the hair cuticles must be well flattened. Raised cuticles lose moisture very fast and this increases porosity and hair toughness. Breakage and weathering of hair is also likely to occur with raised cuticles. Even though hair goes through the usual natural weathering, raised cuticles accelerate the process of weathering. Ceramide oil products act as the cement to prevent all this from happening to the hair cuticles. Other benefits of ceramide oil products are:

- Hair retains moisture

- Restores shine, smoothness and softness to hair
- Improved elasticity and porosity
- Reduces hair loss, fragility, breakage and frizziness of hair
- Protects hair from heat damage from styling and blow dryers
- Can be used to repair hair after chemical processing
- Can be used as often as you wish with quick results
- Can be applied with conditioning treatments

Natural Oils Found in Ceramides

Ceramide products come in two forms. There are those products with natural ingredients and those with synthetic ingredients. Ceramide products with synthetic ingredients more or less mimic the ceramides found inside the cuticles than the natural ceramic products do.

Homemade Ceramide Conditioner Ingredients

If you have the proper ingredients at home, you can easily make your own ceramide conditioner. You do not need to have prior laboratory experience to do this. Home made products have one biggest advantage over all other products bought from stores. They give you the assurance that they are genuinely very natural. You do not have to add any chemicals to enhance color of your hair or increase the products shelf life. You only add what you know your hair needs at that particular time. You also do not need any special equipment to make your own homemade conditioner. You will also cut down on costs by doing this.

Useful Ingredients for Your own DIY Ceramide Formulation

You can have great hair by using simple DIY formulations. Simply buy all the ingredients you need to make your own natural ceramide conditioner. There are many readily available ingredients to make the perfect ceramide conditioner. Some of the natural products you can use to make a great ceramide based hair conditioner that will stick and wash out easily are:

Coconut Milk

Coconut milk is inexpensive and very good for hair that is naturally oily, damaged and dry hair. It is also great for normal and natural hair. Coconut milk can be used with or without any oil to deep condition the hair before washing it. It also helps in clearing up the hair tangles, leaves the hair looking very healthy and rich in volume.

Bananas

Many people may not know the great effects bananas have in conditioning hair. They moisturize and soften the hair. Bananas can be blended together with coconut milk and many other ingredients to give even better results. The mixture is smooth and easy to wash out. It leaves the hair looking very shiny and smooth and strengthens the hair cuticles.

Aloe Vera

Aloe Vera is a widely used ingredient in many products. It can be used in many ways to condition the hair. Use Aloe Vera as a hair spritz made from its juice. This makes a good leave-in-conditioner for the hair. Turn Aloe Vera into a serum to make an easy to use very healthy conditioning serum. Adding Aloe Vera to all your DIY recipes will give the final product more strength and your hair will get a good pH balancing. It also adds more shine to the hair and acts as a great seal to the hair cuticles. Conditioners with Aloe Vera are good for all types of hair and especially quickly repairs any damages caused by chemical hair processors.

Henna

The use of henna on hair leaves it very strong and shiny. Henna conditioners leave lasting effects on the hair. Shinier hair and faster growth are noticeable after a few uses of henna conditioners. Henna effects do not wash away immediately as the henna leaves its deposits into the cuticles. Henna leaves a natural reddish dye on the hair. It does not show much on dark hair tones and for people with blonde hair or light hair colors, it gives red hair highlights.

Cassia Obovata

There is, however, another kind of henna that is colorless Cassia Obovata. Cassia is a neutral henna also used for conditioning and strengthening the hair. It is the best to use because it is neutral. It also gives lighter hair some very beautiful golden highlights. Henna and cassia come in handy in case you want to dye your hair naturally and it covers gray easily and are a good alternative to chemically processed hair dyes.

Vinegar

Vinegar is another product easily found in many homes. It has a natural cleansing and is a very good hair conditioner. Raw unfiltered white and apple cider vinegar is the best vinegar product for the best hair conditioning results. Vinegar can be infused with other natural products to come up with a stronger hair conditioner.

FlaxSeed Oil

Flaxseed oil is a great detangling hair conditioner when infused with other ingredients to moisturize the cuticles as a leave-in-conditioner.

Butter Conditioner

Shea butter and Cocoa butter are natural deep conditioners. Butters are especially good if your hair feels badly dehydrated. Hair butters are also good for braiding hair. The kinds of butter can be mixed with other natural ingredients to make a deep hair conditioner.

Storage

Since you will not be using artificial preservatives you need to take precautions storing your homemade conditioners so they don't ferment or spoil, it is important to use homemade conditioners shortly after you make them but you can refrigerate them for up to a month or freeze single use packets for your following weekly treatments. Oil mixtures are usually fine without refrigeration.

Youthful Hair The Yao Way

The longest hair in the world is a river-side community of women known as the Yao girls. In China's Guangxi there is a mineral-rich river system famous for helping their women to grow long-hair. The Long River is a river system in northern GuangxiProvince, China. It is a part of the larger Pearl River system by way of the Liu, Qian, Xun, and Xi Rivers. The women who wash their hair in this river system are known to have long hair but they have another secret to growing long hair.

The Yao Secret To Long Hair Is Hair Washing With A Fermented Rice Water & Orange Skins Mixture Then Rinsing in Cold River Water.

The Yao secret is their own special hair treatment recipe made of rice water & orange skins that are fermented for a month and applied to their hair as a hair wash for 20 minutes and then rinsing the mixture out in cold river water. All of the women who do this have hair down to their ankles.

Proven Hair Growth Remedies

Studies have been done for the effectiveness of certain substances for hair regrowth. Topical applications of ketoconazole cream, hemp oil, horsetail oil, nettles oil, castor oil, fistril and minoxidil may help with age related hair regrowth.

Nail Rubbing For Hair Growth

This may sound like another fountain of youth myth, but, in Ayurvedic medicine nail rubbing, via pressure points, improves the blood flow to the hair follicle, which strengthens it. Stronger hair follicles drastically reduce hair loss. In fact, after a span of 8 months, hair regrowth is possible. In addition to improving hair quality, rubbing nails to prevent grey hair is a common practice in their culture.

Healthy Nails

The nails can become yellow or brittle with age, also. There is a biofilm beneath the nail bed that can become unhealthy or infected and cause a host of nail problems. Protecting your nails from fungal infection is important as you age. Detoxing your biofilm helps to prevent permanent nail loss. Additionally, a thickening of the nails and yellowish tone is a sign of ill health and sometimes can be associated with aging in older adults.

- Clean under nails daily
- File nails weekly.
- Apply tea tree oil to the nail beds.
- If you work with hands wear gloves
- If you wear polish change it weekly

- Do not wear false nails.
- Avoid mycotoxins and fungal infections

Tips for Stronger Nails

- File snags
- Clip, do not pull off cracked nails
- Take a biotin supplement
- Use caution while nails are soft from water
- Fortify your diet with biotin rich foods
- Be careful about the products you use
- Avoid using acetone, gel and acrylic nails
- Give your nails a break from polish and removers
- Keep your nails ¼ inch or shorter
- Wear cuticle and nail oils to shine

Foods For Strong Nails

Nutrients in food can help your nails become healthier and stronger. Transforming your nails from dry and brittle to healthy and strong can be easy just by changing your diet and grooming habits. Foods that contain keratin building blocks can improve your nails are:

- fruits
- lean meats
- salmon
- leafy greens
- eans
- eggs
- nuts
- whole grains

Chapter 9

Hidden Enemies Of Youthful Vitality

The Hidden Culprits That Accelerate Aging

24 hours a day modern men and women are exposed to environmental and food toxins that many of us don't even realize are there. your body is carrying inflammation and excess toxins and it's not only because of your bad dieting habits or lack of exercise. In fact, it may not even be your fault at all.

Inflammation

Ongoing, chronic inflammation, caused by excess toxins in the body is widespread so you're not alone in this pandemic, it affects millions of Americans and people worldwide. Systemic enzymes play an anti-inflammatory role, simultaneously triggering the rapid removal of cell debris. Given that systemic enzymes are integral in the resolution of fibrin, it's becoming pretty clear that they may be the key to curtailing inflammation in the body and helping to keep your body youthful, vibrant and agile.

Injuries And Prostaglandins

What happens when our body is injured is that it begins to produce certain chemicals called prostaglandins. A specific form of prostaglandin causes inflammation. The result of this is swelling, constriction of blood vessels and decreased tissue permeability. Systemic enzymes help by breaking down these proteins in traumatized tissue.

Silent Killers

We're exposed to so many hidden toxins that get into our bodies that work our immune systems into exhaustion. Many of those toxins are hidden silent killers, some are still unknown to us. But most are *avoidable* when you know *what* they are and *where* they are coming from.

Consequences of Inflammation

Our modern lives bring into our bodies amounts of toxic materials that we often just can't deal with which means the immune system's work is never-ending. There's little let-up in the excess toxins it's forced to deal with and on constant high-alert and always being called into action it becomes stressed and exhausted and at times experiences a burn-out of sorts. Which leads to it making some serious internal signalling mistakes, most notably it sends inflammatory cells everywhere – and they start to attack healthy body tissue and whatever tissue they attack leads to a specific disease. This is called an immune system disorder. In fact, scientists have verified over a hundred immune system disorders. They take different forms, attacking different parts of the body.

- In rheumatoid arthritis, the immune system is attacking your joints and connective tissues.
- In diabetes, it is attacking your pancreas.
- In celiac disease it's attacking your gut lining.
- In Hashimoto's thyroiditis, the victims are your thyroid cells.

Solutions For Lowering Inflammation

There are specific substances that help with lowering inflammatory responses and some others that help the body to detox and eliminate existing inflammation.

- **Glucosamine**

    Glucosamine is a substance that keeps the connective tissues of your body strong and healthy therefore, supplements containing glucosamine are effective for anti-aging. Glucosamine helps in the regeneration of of your digestive tract and also skin cells so that old and worn out cells that give the skin a dull appearance are replaced by new cells, for healthier and younger skin. This cell renewal process helps by replacing old, dead, dull skin with new skin that has fewer signs of aging. Glucosamine helps in the exfoliation of skin and can even help reverse wrinkles and fine lines that already present on the face or scarring in your gut lining from food allergies such as those with a gluten allergy.

- **Carnosine**

    Carnosine is an amino acid combination of alanine and histidine, taking it in supplement form is a very effective anti-aging compound. Carnosine itself is a compound that inhibits the breakdown of proteins in the skin. This includes collagen and other proteins that are essential for the vitality of the skin. It reduces the chances of premature aging. It is one of the anti-oxidants that fights free radicals and prevents them from damaging the skin. It is important that you maintain smart dietary and lifestyle habits to achieve successful reverse aging. Just remember that it is the biological clock we are trying to manipulate and not the chronological one.

Chapter 10

Hidden Toxins Health Destroyers

Avoid Environmental Toxins In Your Home Or Place Of Work

It is important to be aware of seemingly harmless toxins that can be invisible health and beauty destroyers in your environment. A few that come to mind are:

- Radon Gas
- Asbestos
- Toxic Mold
- Carbon Monoxide
- And more...

It is a good idea to have your home tested yearly and if you have gas leaks, water leaks, roof or foundation cracks or water damage problems you may have invisible health hazards that should be repaired by a professional, promptly. Even during basic housekeeping always wear a mask and gloves when cleaning or dusting under cabinets, beds, furniture closets, garages, sheds or when cleaning outdoor patios and pool houses because there can be dangerous mold or dust present especially in older homes or water damaged buildings. Mycotoxins are health and beauty destroyers, they damage cells, age your skin quickly and can lead to severe internal health damage that rob you of youthful vitality.

Additionally, if you have leaks get them repaired and cleaned by a professional if there are signs of water damage, call mold remediation experts, immediately. Mold produces mycotoxins that can make you very sick by breathing the spores or even touching them through the skin and lungs. Do not take a risk with your health, mycotoxins can ruin your health for a very long time and some people can even die from it. If you think you may have been exposed do not hesitate to have a urine mycotoxin test, if you doctor won't order a mycotoxin test find a doctor or health provider who will. Most blood and urine tests do not check mycotoxin levels; a specific test for mycotoxin levels must be examined. Other health hazards can come from mouse or insect droppings. To make it simple it is very important to keep an extremely clean living environment and shelter that keeps out all outside elements effectively.

How toxins damage our bodies

Basically, there are eight ways toxins damage our bodies.

Toxins poison enzymes so they don't work properly.

Our bodies are enzyme engines. Every physiological function depends on enzymes to manufacture molecules, produce energy, and create cell structures. Toxins damage enzymes and thus undermine countless bodily functions inhibiting the production of hemoglobin in the blood, for example, or lowering the body's capacity to prevent the free-radical damage that accelerates aging.

Toxins Displace Structural Minerals

People need to maintain healthy bone mass for lifelong mobility. When toxins displace the calcium present in bone, there is a twofold effect: weaker skeletal structures and increased toxins, released by bone loss, which circulates throughout the body.

Toxins Damage The Organs

Toxins damage nearly all your organs and systems. My book, The Toxin Solution, focuses specifically on the detox organs. If your digestive tract, liver, and kidneys are so toxic they are unable to detox effectively, your detoxification will backfire and your body will remain toxic.

Toxins Damage DNA & Accelerate Aging

Toxins increase the rate of aging and degeneration. Many commonly used pesticides, phthalates, improperly detoxified estrogens, and products containing benzene damage DNA.

Toxins modify gene expression.

Our genes switch off and on to adapt to changes in our bodies and the outer environment. But many toxins activate or suppress our genes in undesirable ways.

Toxins Damage Cell Membranes

"Signaling" in the body happens in the cell membranes. Damage to these membranes prevent them from getting important messages such as:

- Insulin not signaling the cells to absorb so you lose energy
- Muscle cells not responding to the message from magnesium so you lose strength
- Muscles lose cell signals to relax resulting in pain and many various problems from muscle spasms to heart attacks depending on the severity of the toxic exposure.

Toxins Cause Hormone Imbalances.

Toxins induce, inhibit, mimic, and block hormones. One example: Arsenic disrupts thyroid hormone receptors on the cells, so the cells don't get the message from the thyroid hormones that cause them to rev up metabolism. The result is inexplicable fatigue.

Toxins Impair Your Ability To Detoxify

When you are very toxic and desperately need to detoxify, it's harder to do than when you are *not* toxic. In other words, just when you need your detox systems most, your hard-working detox system is most likely to be functioning below par. Why? Because the heavy toxic load you already carry has overwhelmed your detox capacity. That's right. The more toxins you have burdening your body, the greater the damage to your body's detoxification pathways. That's why restoring your detox organs and with them your detox pathways is such an important challenge. The net result is that you can readily release toxins from your body.

Food Lectin Precautions

Lectins, a type of carbohydrate-binding protein found in most types of beans and lentils and some other foods. Lectins stick to cell membranes in the digestive tract. They exist in most plant and animal foods. However, they're found in the highest amounts in:

- Legumes
- Nightshade vegetables
- Dairy products
- Grains, such as:

    o barley
    o quinoa
    o rice

There's limited research on how lectins affect people. The lectin-free diet promotes reducing intake of or completely eliminating lectins from your diet. This may be beneficial for some people with food sensitivities. However, more research is still needed.

Ricin Food Toxin

Some types of lectins, such as ricin, are toxic and are found in some foods such as:

- Castor beans
- Castor oil

Hazardous Ricin In Food: Just one castor bean has enough Ricin to kill a child, and just a few more can kill an adult. A single gram of ricin, the bean's main toxin, is thousands of times more powerful than cyanide but it is destroyed during washing, soaking, cooking or heating.

Lectins Are Bad For You

Studies show that lectins are found in 30% of the food we eat. For most people, if these foods are cooked properly, they do not give you health problems. Soaking the bean in water can eliminate much of the lectin since lectin is water-soluble. Additionally, the heat generated during the cooking process destroys most lectins.

On the other hand, if you have food sensitivities or are prone to gastrointestinal distress, avoiding foods with lectins may be beneficial. Lectins haven't been studied extensively in humans. Currently, there's no evidence that concludes whether it's good or bad for your health. The lectin-free diet is restrictive and eliminates many nutrient-dense foods even those thought to be healthy.

Effects Of Lectin

Lectins may affect people with food sensitivities and those with thyroid issues. Eating large amounts of food containing lectins may cause thyroid imbalances, gas or gastric distress in some people. For some, lectins are not digestible. Lectins bind to the cell membranes that make up the lining of the digestive tract and they may disrupt metabolism and cause damage to this lining.

Lectins Can Be Potentially Toxic

Cooking destroys most lectins in your food. It's important to avoid raw, soaked, or undercooked beans, such as kidney beans, which have been found to be toxic to people due to their lectin levels. Studies show that soaking beans isn't enough to remove lectin content. They must be cooked to reduce the lectin in them research shows that lectins can disrupt digestion, interfere with nutrient absorption and cause intestinal damage if eaten in large quantities over a prolonged period of time.

Chapter 11

Anti Aging Beauty Treatments

There is a glow that is associated with youth. We've all heard of that "youthful glow". The energy in the body is highest when we are young and that energy is instantly noticeable and there are ways to keep it from fading with age for example, by taking a cell energy supercharger, such as an AMPK boosters. There is also a glow that comes with self-confidence and self-love that is also very attractive. Keeping your energies up is a sign of youthful vitality and many beauty treatments can help you keep that youthful glow.

The most beautiful people take good care of their appearance

Beautiful Smile

The most important thing to wear is a smile. A smile can help you look years younger, too. Keep your teeth bright and your lips moist. Use tooth whitening products. Keep your breath fresh. Do things that make you happy and that keep a smile on your face. Happy, feel-good hormones are great for anti-aging, too. As far as your skin goes, it is most important to keep your skin clean, exfoliated and moisturized.

Enzyme Scrub Up

Exfoliating twice a week is an excellent way to stimulate your cells' renewal and activity. By removing the dead cells at the surface, the skin will find a balance to stimulate the renewal. Use fruit enzymes instead of harsh nut shell fiber. The alpha hydroxy acids in fruits also help your skin glow, too.

Hydration & Moisturizing

Since dehydration is our skin's worst enemy. Hydration is important from drinking enough water daily to bathing and applying moisturisers. H2o is important because it not only hydrates our body and skin while we bathe, internally, water is a source of internal oxygen that keeps cells healthy and revitalized, replenishing our inner fountain of youth.

Drinking Water Replenishes Your Inner Fountain Of Youth.

Activate Fountain Of Youth In Your Skin

Essential oils and hydrating sprays are the best natural substances to help give your skin that youthful glow.

- Ceramide face spray (rice ceramide water)
- Placenta face cream (stem cell renewal)
- Buchinol oil (natural retin-a without the irritation)
- Frankincense oil (natural anti-wrinkle)
- Pacholli oil (natural skin tightener)

Get Your Beauty Sleep

No, it's not just an old wives' tale – sleep really does make you look young and beautiful as it's the time when your cells are most active. As Dr. Neuser explains, "Sleep deprivation does not just mean dark circles, puffiness, and breakouts. When you're sleepy, chances are that your skin is feeling it too. This means that your skin produces less chemical energy, which slows down cell regeneration and vital skin processes such as repair from UV and environmental damage."

Cleopatra's Beauty Secrets

Cleopatra is known to have been one of the earliest seeker's of the fountain of youth. There were several beauty practices that Cleopatra followed consistently, everyday to cultivate her beauty. These tips are simple enough that every woman could do them.

- Milk and honey bath - for soft, healthy and glowing skin
- Almond oil- she used almond oil as a moisturizer
- Sea salt scrub- she did salt body scrubs to exfoliate
- Rose water toner- she splashed rose water on to hydrate
- Beeswax face cream- she used a night cream
- Natural shampoo- she used henna for shiny hair
- She used soured milk - lactic acid mask for smooth skin
- Eyeshadow- green malachite or blue lapis paste on her lids.
- Lipstick and rouge- she used red ochre clay with iron oxide.
- Eyeliner- she used Khol as black eyeliner, brows and lashes.

Best Home Beauty Treatments

- **Derma Roller**

  A derma-roller facial causes trauma to the skin, which then stimulates new collagen to help it refresh and look plumper. It helps remove stretch marks, refreshes sun-damaged skin and reduces fine lines and wrinkles. This treatment has an immediate effect and as the serums start to work over the coming weeks, it only gets better.

Facial Mesotherapy

This facial treats the skin from the inside out. Using micro injections, helps insert nutrients, vitamins and minerals into the middle layer (epidermis) of the skin to rejuvenate it. It tightens natural sagging, improves the appearance of wrinkles and can restructure mature skin to leave it firmer. You will see smoother skin immediately and the results will continue to increase. If you book three or more appointments, these results will continue to get better and better.

TCA, Glycolic & Lactic Acid Skin Peel

This treatment is for anyone wishing to reveal plumper, younger looking skin. It doesn't have to be for your face either. You can use this on your neck, chest, arms or hands. Anywhere that you'd like to refresh the appearance of the skin.

Urotherapy

People applying urine to their faces. These skin peels contain a form of uric or lactic acid that helps to remove the dead skin cells. Fresh skin cells are then produced, leaving you with fresher and brighter skin.

Microcurrent & Natural Face Lift Options

If you don't want to have any chemical treatments at all, this is the perfect solution. Perfect for relaxing tension and the muscles in the face and neck, it releases toxins, leaving you with a visibly refreshed stress-free face. Including Japanese facial massage, acupuncture and facial techniques, wrinkles are reduced and you get an instant face lift. All without any painful surgery. Perfect.

Anti-Aging Facial Yoga For Forehead:

- Smooth Vertical "11" between the brow
- Smooth "Thinker-Lines" Worry lines
- Smooth Horizontal Forehead Lines

Good For Preventing:

- Horizontal forehead lines.
- Alternative To: Botox

Step 1

Place both hands on the forehead facing inwards and spread all of the fingers out between the eyebrows and hairline.

Step 2

Gently sweep the fingers outwards across the forehead, applying light pressure to tighten the skin.

Step 3

Relax and repeat 10 times.

Facial Expression Awareness Exercise

Tape a piece of sports tape between the brow and crow's feet, learn the moods and emotions that cause you to wrinkle between your eyebrows. Over time this will help you prevent making wrinkle-causing facial expression lines that show up as wrinkling your forehead and around your eyes.

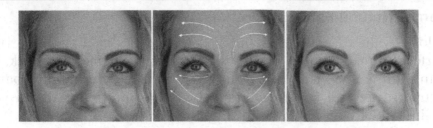

Brow Lift Exercise & Anti-Aging Benefits For Eyes:

On a nightly basis after removing your makeup, apply face-lift oil to fingertips, lightly massage into your skin according to the direction of the arrows above avoiding eye area.

1. Lift brow muscles upward then relax brow muscle.
2. Repeat quickly 10 times.
3. Repeat 3 sets of 10, nightly.

Benefits:

- Lifts the brow
- Improves Dull Skin
- Improves Blood flow and glow.
- Improves Dark Circles
- Decreases Puffy Eyes
- Lifts Drooping eyebrows
- Lifts Sagging cheeks
- Smooths Forehead wrinkles

Oooh-La-La Face Lift Exercise

The Oooh-La-La face exercise helps lift the lower jowl and neck, it also improves upper body posture. It is greatly beneficial for those with the loose skin under the chin, commonly known as "turkey-neck". It is a quick, effective and easy daily exercise that can be done in less than 5 minutes each day that will help keep you looking younger for many years to come. Most healthy people can do this but if you have neck or back problems ask your doctor first. Here's how to do it.

Instructions:

- Sit or stand with a straight spine
- Roll shoulders back
- Push chest outward
- Slowly tilt head back
- Looking up toward the sky
- Pucker lips without wrinkling them and say Ooooh
- Smile show teeth and say La La
- Oooh La La, Oooh La La, Oooh La La!
- Repeat 10 Times

  - Optional- with or without raised arms to work trapezius and back neck muscles which gives a more defined lift.

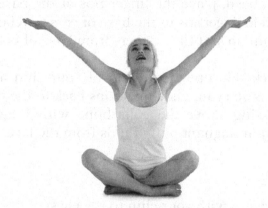

Kiss The Sky Exercise For Neck:

- Tilt head back, pucker and kiss toward the sky, repeat ten times daily.
- Good For: Lines and loose skin on the neck.
- Alternative To: Neck or jowl lift.

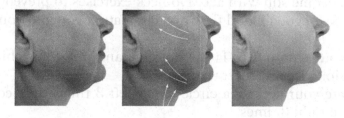

Drain Stagnant Fluid Buildup & Lift Sagging Facial Muscles

Step 1

- Make a peace-sign with your middle and index fingers
- Place your fingertips above and below your cheekbone.
- Push facial tissues up to the top of the ears with the 2 fingertips and then gently over the ear, behind the ear and down to the base of your neck at the collar bone.
- Looking straight ahead, place the finger tips at the base of the collarbone and pump with light presses to drain lymph.
- Repeat 3 times.

Step 2

- Looking straight ahead, place the finger tips at the base of the back of your neck and skull, glide fingertips to the base of ears to relax tension.
- Tilt head back, chin up and flide fingers from base of collarbone up to the tip of the chin.
- Lightly stroke neck skin upwards to tip of your chin as you tilt your head backwards as far as you can, glide fingertips back to the base of the collarbone while gently pressing above the collarbone with fingertips in a pumping motion to help drain stagnant puffy fluids from the face.

Step 3

- Tilt your head forward with your chin to the chest.
- Looking straight ahead, place the finger tips at the bottom of the collarbone and lightly stroke the skin upwards to stimulate blood flow to the face and restore a healthy glow.

Step 4

- Our joints become stiff with age. Do neck exercises to prevent loss of mobility and to help keep good blood flow and circulation going to your head and face.
    - Jut your chin out as far as possible and pull your chin back as far as possible. Repeat several times.
    - Rotate your neck in a circle to the left 3 times then counter-clockwise to the right 3 times.

Step 5

- Drain your facial lymphatics. Place your fingertips under the base of your collarbone
- Press fingertips gently into the groove above the collarbone, tilt head back and point your chin upwards.
- Pump the fingertips to drain lymphatics and pump away stagnant fluids, this will help drain inflammation from the face and help eliminate puffy tired skin.

Take three deep breaths. Repeat 3 times.

You can do these therapies on yourself or have a friend or therapist to do it for you. It is a fun practice for couples, too.

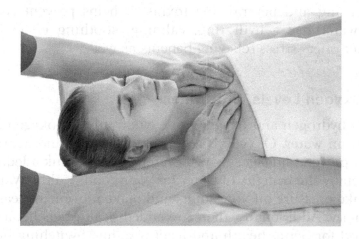

Massage & Touch Therapy

Therapeutic touch therapy (TT) increased the level of blood hemoglobin and hematocrit, significantly. Massage therapy (MT) also increases the levels of hemoglobin which stimulates all self-healing mechanisms in the body.

Sound Therapy Binaural Beats

Some health practitioners believe that there are healing frequencies and sounds. Soothing sounds can help reduce stress, upbeat sounds can improve mood and a better sense of joy. While harsh loud sounds can be annoying and stressing and some very high decibels are known to shatter glass. Therefore, it is worth having a look into sound therapy and its many benefits for anti-aging.

Water Therapy Exercises

Water is cleansing, refreshing, relaxing, revitalising and invigorating, depending on the temperature or flow of the water you are submersed in. A bath can calm you down, a cold water-fall can invigorate you. Drinking water is also an important part of life as our body's are over 70% water. Everyone knows about the importance of good hygiene. It's important to:

- Wash our hands frequently and
- Bathe or shower daily
- Drink plenty of water daily
- Do water exercises, when you exercise in water it is a type of resistance training which strengthens your muscles without adding pressure on your joints.

Water is cleansing and neutralizing toxins, it helps prevent risk of infectious conditions and water has a hydrating, calming, soothing effect in many ways. Additionally, water offers stress relieving benefits as well.

Increase Your Oxygen Levels With Water

Water is H2O hydrogen and oxygen. So we not only get oxygen from the air we breath we get it from water. Oxygen is a nutrient the brain and heart need constant flow of oxygen to prevent damage. As you exercise more, drink adequate amounts of water, daily and enjoy the benefits of water for your good-health. Water aerobics and water exercises take pressure off your joints and make movements easier without the full weight of gravity. Additionally, there are added health benefits as contrast baths are especially good for better health and healthy aging. Switching between hot and cold water stimulates many natural healing mechanisms within the body. Finish off every shower or bath with a cool water rinse and the colder you can tolerate it the better for toning the tissues over time it helps keep your body firmer. Exfoliating and Body brushing also helps with cell renewal and circulation and are a healthy hygiene exercise to include in your daily self-care routine.

Water Therapy Calms The Mind & Body

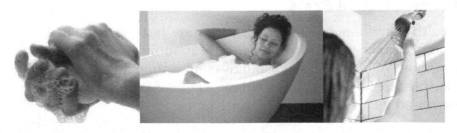

Water Therapy Benefits

Water is the most important substance that we consume. In Ayurveda, the original Mind-Body medicine was water treatments. Experts suggest that you must drink water first thing in the morning as it plays a key role in boosting your overall health. There are other morning rituals that are recommended before eating any food such as oil pulling which involves swishing and gargling with a special blend of Ayurvedic oils and tongue brushing to remove film and mucus.

In Japan, water therapy is the first morning ritual and it is said to help relieve stress, promote weight loss and strengthen the digestive system. Most of all, it gives you energy throughout the day. Additionally, drinking water during the day also helps boost your metabolism. For those who are suffering from health conditions or those who are beginners, begin water therapy with one glass of water and gradually increase water intake. In Japan, it is believed that water therapy can help to cure a variety of diseases.

The Five Steps Of Japanese Water Therapy Are:

1. Water- First step, when you wake up in the morning, is to drink three 10 oz glasses of water on an empty stomach. The water should be at room temperature or lukewarm.

    o (may add lemon)

2. Oral Hygiene- Brush your teeth after drinking water with ginger or mint water.

    o (may add baking soda)

3. Morning Water Fast- Avoid eating or drinking anything for at least 30-40 minutes.

    o (may afterwards have your usual green tea or coffee)

4. Portion Control- After each meal, do not eat or drink anything else

    o (wait at least two hours before eating anything else).

5. Breaking A Fast- Drink water and tea.

Water is actually a means of giving the body more oxygen and drinking water is an important part of every fit and healthy lifestyle and a necessary part of your daily longevity routine.

Other Japanese good health practices:

- Walk every day for at least an hour. This helps in speeding up your metabolism.
- Choose a lovely place for your daily walk such as a Japanese garden, a bamboo forest, a babbling brook or a beach, walk with intent and quietly be at one with nature. Primordial sounds of the wilderness bring a greater sense of peace and wellness.
- Each night, before bed, gargle a few times with warm salt water for a few minutes then spit it out.
- Do not eat or drink while standing, be seated and practice mindful eating.
- Chew your food properly before swallowing it down as it helps produce digestive enzymes and aids in better digestion of food and absorption of nutrients.
- Drink hot water with mint, lemon or green tea.

Used Tea Bag Home Treatments

Before you throw your tea bags or loose tea grounds away! Save them to add to you your smoothies or for beauty treatments. The added antioxidants are very beneficial for your skin and are a good anti-aging home remedy.

- After a wet bag is cool, wipe the moist bag over your face, decollete and whole body.
- Add the contents of one tea bag to your smoothie recipe
- Drop a few used tea bags in a tea bath
- Add used tea bags to your foot bath
- Add to body scrub
- Add to body wash
- Apply the cooled grounds directly to thighs and wrap in cellophane for a home cellulite treatment.
- Use the cool grounds as a compress on mosquito bites, minor stings or minor burns.

Sea Salt

Sea salt is hailed for its health-enhancing minerals, therapeutic properties, and all-natural harvesting process. Adding a little sea salt to your bath can help:

- Stimulate circulation,
- Ease muscle cramps,
- Help relieve stiffness in joints,
- Aid with arthritis or
- Alleviate back pain, and
- Soothe achy legs and feet.

There are a myriad of reasons to incorporate salt baths into your routine.

- **Builds Immunity** - Soaking in sea salt baths on a regular basis is beneficial as we expose ourselves to highly absorptive minerals that boost our resistance to illness and disease. Similar to the effects of physical exercise, warm baths have also been found to trigger an anti-inflammatory response that is vital for increasing our body's ability to ward off diseases and illness. There is also an immune-boosting effect of the salt baths. High in antibacterial properties, the soak helps eliminate pathogens while staving off harmful microbes.
- **Increases Energy** - When our bodies are not getting the minerals they need, fatigue begins to set in. Magnesium, in particular, is important for managing our stress response, but unfortunately, 57% of adults do not meet their recommended magnesium intake. This deficiency can lead to disrupted sleep and muscle fatigue. By indulging in a Salt Soak, you can restore the energy in your cells and make your way to a revitalized self.
- **Balances Chemistry Adds Alkalinity**- Excess acidity in the body from an improper diet can lead to overworking of our vital organs, which then must take minerals from our bones and tissue. The baking soda in our salt soaks is a naturally alkaline substance with a reputation for removing toxins effectively. Introducing salt soaks to your life is a great way to remove excess acid from the cells and reintroduce trace minerals back into your body.
- **Soothes Muscle Injury** - Being in a warm bath can ease pain by taking the weight off joints and muscles. It can also help your body to heal faster after an injury or surgery. When used with warm water, the magnesium-rich salt helps relieve muscle spasms and menstrual cramps. We love the idea of settling into a bath with our Bath Salt after a hard workout or a long day for indulgent relief.
- **Promotes Restful Sleep** - A warm salt bath is perfect for helping us relax when we're anxious or tense. The temperature changes your body goes through when switching from a warm bath to cooler air can actually help

improve sleep. In addition, the proper ratio of water and salt exposure can help prevent the need to urinate during the night, leading to less disrupted sleep. The Good Night Bath Saltis packed with ultra-relaxing essential oils like Lavender and Chamomile to enhance your nighttime sleep routine.

- **Improves Skin Health** - The minerals inside a high-quality salt soak promote healthy, more youthful skin. When we emerge from the water, our skin is left silky and smooth. Salt soaks also help purge impurities from the skin and balances skin moisture levels. The use of dead sea salts has also been implemented for the treatment of psoriasis. Not only is salt good for dry, itchy skin and acne, but research also suggests that the baking soda in salt soaks may be useful as an antifungal agent for skin and nails.

- **Decreases Congestion** - Allergies and infections can lead to a buildup of mucus, which everyone has to cope with at one time or another. Not only does a salt bath help to eliminate existing mucus buildup, but it can also help to prevent it. The eucalyptus cardamom bath salt includes eucalyptus essential oil, which works alongside the nutrient-dense salts to actively help decongest the respiratory system.

- **Aids in Chronic Pain Relief** - While we may not be able to free ourselves from chronic pain, we can soothe our bodies in a nourishing salt bath. Warm water baths are highly effective at treating lower back pain, and dead sea salts have been utilized for the treatment of rheumatoid arthritis.

- **Boosts Overall Health** - Studies show that these baths can improve our health in general. Benefits range from regulating blood sugar and improving cardiovascular health, to boosting circulatory and nerve function. We suggest pairing the natural healing qualities of a warm salt bath with aromatherapy for further rejuvenation. A Grapefruit Pink Pepper Bath Salt is particularly effective at supporting the lymphatic system and fighting free radicals.

- **Because They Feel Good!**- Not only is salt soaks healing for the body, but they are also so beneficial to our mental wellbeing. Don't just take a bath because you need it, take one because you want to. Tangerine Jasmine Bath Salt is for those times when you just need to treat yourself. Sit back, relax, and indulge in the restorative properties of Epsom and sea salts and the therapeutic benefits of 100% pure essential oils.

Cleansing Enema

The purpose of the enema is to cleanse the colon, blood and clear the liver of toxins. These toxins occur from the normal metabolisms of food as well as the carcinogenic toxins from our polluted environment, drugs, food and water pollutants such as pesticides, preservatives, hormones, excreted prescription drugs and fluoride.

Home Colon Cleansing Mechanisms

This cleansing is accomplished by increasing the liver's capacity to detoxify toxins in the blood and binding them to the bile. In the process, the liver cleanses itself as it releases the toxic bile into the small, then large, intestine for evacuation. The entire blood supply circulates through the liver every three minutes. By retaining the coffee 12 to 15 minutes, the blood will circulate four to five times for cleansing, much like a dialysis treatment. The water content of the coffee stimulates intestinal peristalsis and helps to empty the large intestine with the accumulated toxic bile. Coffee enemas are not primarily for colon cleansing it is more for liver cleansing and to increase glutathione.

Homemade Saline Enema Recipe

You can make a homemade saline solution:

- 1 Quart Distilled Water
- 2 level teaspoons of table salt to a quart of lukewarm distilled water.
- **Do not use:**

  o soapsuds,
  o hydrogen peroxide, or
  o tap water as an enema. They have contaminants that may be dangerous.

Weight Loss Fiber & Colon Cleansing

Fiber is in the peel and rind of many fruits and vegetables, many people throw the fiber part of their food away. But Fiber offers many benefits. Eating more soluble fiber can also help you lose belly fat and prevent belly fat gain. One study linked a 10-gram increase in daily soluble fiber intake to a 3.7% lower risk of gaining belly fat. Several other studies also show that people who eat more soluble fiber have a lower risk of belly fat. You will know if you are getting enough dietary fiber by the weight and bulk of your stool, it should float and if it does you're getting enough fiber. If not, take a daily fiber supplement and watch belly fat fade away in a few months.

Glutathione Physiology

Glutathione is the primary antioxidant that is prevalent in every cell in the human body. Glutathione is primarily synthesized in the liver where it is abundantly present. Glutathione participates in leukotriene synthesis for WBC mobilization and is a

119

cofactor for the enzyme glutathione peroxidase, a powerful cellular antioxidant. There are few sources to help increase these nutrients in your body:

- **Caffeine**- palmitic acid in caffeine increases the activity of glutathione S-transferase (GST) by 600% in the liver and a 700% increase in detoxification in the small intestine.
- **Cruciferous Vegetables**- GST(glutathione S-transferase) makes excess free radicals water soluble for easy elimination from the cells and the body and blocks and detoxifies carcinogens. GST, binds bilirubin and its glucuronides so that they can be eliminated from the hepatocytes (liver cells).

The liver uses glutathione to neutralize poisons, alcohol, caffeine, medications, nicotine, and remove them from your blood and helps your body maintain homeostasis. The amino acid, Cysteine is the limiting factor as (NAC) N-acetyl-Cysteine is used in glutathione synthesis.

An adequate supply of Glutathione helps cleanse your blood of toxins.

90% of the blood supply to the stomach and intestines passes through the liver. The blood carries important nutrients to the liver where they are metabolized into substances vital to life preserving detoxification processes. When toxic substances reach the liver they are activated or transformed into less toxic derivatives. Glutathione plays a crucial role in the processes of the liver's detoxification and biotransformation systems. Biotransformation in Phase One denatures toxins and Phase Two transmutates toxins into a water soluble form that helps to bind toxins with bile and excrete the toxins out of your body through the feces.

Drug Use Colon Cleansing
People who take narcotic barbiturates are often constipated as the drugs are antispasmodic and interfere with peristaltic action and enemas help generate bowel movements.

Enemas To Alleviate Drug Induced Constipation

Dr. Gerson, MD was a pioneer in colon cleansing and recommended that his drug addicted patients use coffee enemas to remove morphine and relieve their severe pain. However, people who use narcotic medications should consult with their primary doctor if they are experiencing constipation.

Coffee Enemas Summary:

- Cleanses the blood of toxins
- Cleanses the liver to improve its many metabolic functions
- Boost the immune system
- Relieves severe pain and some headaches

Accumulated toxins have been associated with general nervous tension, confusion, depression, allergy related symptoms and severe pain.

How To Do Enemas & Colon Cleansing

You can buy enema kits over the counter. When preparing to take the enema, it is best to empty the colon first and follow the manufacturer's directions on the label. For more information and techniques about home colon cleansing search online and ask your health professional for specific instructions.

3 Minute Mind Calming Exercise

Think of the beauty of nature, a gentle stream, a beautiful beach, a field of wildflowers, if you can go take a walk in a place like this, even better, but if not you can always go there in your mind and the calming effects are similar according to brain scientists. For those who can't venture outdoors you can calm your mind anywhere, anyplace and anytime by simply doing the following.

Sit in a quiet and comfortable place. Put one of your hands on your chest and the other on your stomach.

1. Close your eyes, relax your body and mind.
2. Begin to relax by breathing deeply and slowly
3. Inhale- Take long slow deep breaths and regular breath in through your nose.
4. Exhale- Breathe out through your mouth, slowly and completely.
5. Calm your mind, and relax more deeply, take your thoughts off of daily life and imagine yourself in a tranquil place.

6. Repeat this process at least 10 times or until you begin to feel stress and anxiety subside.

Think of nature, a gentle stream, a beautiful beach, a field of wildflowers, if you can go take a place like this, even better but if not you can always go there in your mind and the calming effects are similar according to brain scientists.

Massages Boost Blood Circulation

Massages aren't just great for your body, but for your face too especially when it comes to anti-aging. "Massaging the face and more specifically the areas where you see wrinkles and loss of firmness is very important. Massaging helps to activate the blood circulation, so your anti-aging cream is much more easily absorbed by the skin. Moreover, the massage helps to stimulate the synthesis of collagen in the skin as it improves the intercellular connections. That's why pinching and tapping the skin helps the blood to come up to the surface, which also boosts radiance!

Move More

Getting regular physical activity activates the blood circulation and oxygenation of the body, and makes you sweat. This will help detoxify the skin to give you better cell activity.

Age Related Brain Fitness and Exercises

Declining brain health and memory loss are not inevitable parts of aging! You can be mentally sharp and maintain your ability to learn, reason, and remember into old age by eating right, exercising your mind and body, getting enough sleep, managing stress, connecting with others, and challenging your brain.

- Read & Recall Exercise- Reading is an activity that boosts cognitive skills and enhances lost vocabulary, reading can help reduce feelings of isolation for anyone anywhere anytime. I can help elderly enhance memory so ask your older loved one to retell the story they read once they have finished each chapter in the book to increase social interactions with each other.
- Reading and storytelling is a brain exercise that helps us develop sharper memory skills.
- Practice happy outcome storytelling.
- Sing songs, it stimulates your brain to remember the words and tones.
- Repeat the lyrics and do a voice scale of the musical notes, tones and sounds.

- High blood sugar is linked to memory loss
- Your diet and exercise practices can help you fight against the brain changes linked to dementia and Alzheimer's disease
- Deep sleep may help wash away beta-amyloid plaques linked to Alzheimer's disease
- Certain exercise lower your risk of dementia and helps boosts new neuron development
- Eat a brain-boosting diet, eat more good fats and avoid processed sugar.
- Do exercises that help improve cognitive fitness
- Drink camomile tea before bed to improve sleep
- Do deep breathing techniques to manage stress
- Stay socially active
- Do activities to challenge your brain such as puzzles and games
- Younger teens may prefer VR and video games
- Children and elderly can name things you can wear on your feet that start with the letter "s"
- Play trivia games, checkers, dominos, cards, board games, ect.
- Name an object for every alphabet in your name. Over time, work up to naming 3 or more objects or words that start with each letter of your name, try using different words each time.
- Take a course, learn something, new.
- Pick a new topic to study.
- Keep your mind active, too.

Chapter 12

Anti Aging Diet & Nutrition Tips

Good nutrition is important as the foods we eat feed our inner fountain of youth. Our body needs the daily recommended allowance of nutrients to function properly and for hunger to be satisfied. Additionally, our body requires a daily intake of adequate amounts of water, typically, our body weight, divided in half equals the number of ounces of water we need to drink in a day. In times of stress, we produce adrenaline and other harmful stress hormones causing a need for extra nutrition, as stress burns up B vitamins and depletes our adrenals which can cause us to crave carbs and sugar for fuel while slowing down our metabolism and causing our body to store more fat.

The Effects of Stress Eating

Stress burns up our vitamin B reserves and then we can suffer from adrenal burn out as a side effect. The body can not distinguish between psychological and physiological stress, it treats both types of stress the same way. Too much stress puts the body into fight-or-flight mode, pulling blood flow away from the organ systems and when we are in that mode our metabolism slows down and since we are not digesting, we could be gaining unwanted weight. Sometimes during times of stress. Luckily, there are plenty of foods rich in B vitamins. Good sources include wholegrain cereals, meat, poultry, eggs, nuts, fish, milk, legumes and fresh vegetables.

Calming Cravings & A Voracious Appetite

When we exercise it stimulates our appetite. If we are not getting enough minerals and amino-acids for muscle fuel we will experience excessive hunger. Sometimes even if we are not hungry we have cravings and that can be a simple fix, it is likely that you are not getting enough minerals if you crave salt or crunch snacks. We have 5 types of taste-bud senses that need daily satisfaction, sweet, salty, sour, bitter and spicy hot. If you crave spicy food you likely need more zinc. If spicy foods seem too hot you likely have enough zinc. Zinc and magnesium are synergistic and if you get too much of one you can't absorb the other. Zinc is the energy conductor in the body. The body uses **zinc** to process nutrients. Make sure you get all the flavors daily and your appetite and your taste buds will be more satisfied with your diet. Go for lower calorie foods with high water content that are more filling, broths, salads and whole fruits such as grapefruit. Avoid processed foods empty of nutrition and filled with preservatives, excess salt, sugar and fat. Also, greatly limit foods such as cheese, pasta and bread. However, a very small half-portion is better than feeling deprived.

Portion Control

Portion size and portion control are the two most important factors. Too much of a good thing can make you fat. Moderation is key for everything in life and especially food. Always eat a normal size portion and remember your stomach is only about the size of your fist the more you stretch it the harder it is to control your appetite and feel full eating a normal sized portion. Overeating is never good.

Hot Drinks

Having a hot drink can jump start metabolism. Soothe and calm stress and has a whole host of other benefits depending on the type of hot drink you choose. Hot drinks and beverages such as green tea, hot chocolate, and coffee are frequently served at temperatures between 160 degrees F or 71.1 degrees celsius because brief exposures to liquids in this temperature range can cause significant scald burns and you should allow your hot drink to cool to a temperature below 120 degrees fahrenheit or 65 degrees celcius before drinking it.

Microwave, Boiling & Heating

Microwaving any foods or liquids is not an anti-aging practice, ever as it produces cancer-causing acrylamides in all liquids including water.

Cooking

Anytime we want to change the molecular structure of something in a laboratory, we heat it up. The same thing happens when we heat foods. When you cook veggies, the heat kills enzymes. Enzymes are important for every function in your body. Never microwave it alters your food's chemistry in a negative way that can cause harm. Microwaving is an absolute, no-no, microwaving creates known carcinogens called acrylamides in food and beverages. Avoid burning food when cooking, as burning processed meats that are loaded with preservatives, also causes carcinogens to form in your food. Sure have some cooked foods, but let raw, organic non-gmo foods dominate your diet.

Diet & Nutrition

Getting enough proper good nutrition is important. Our body requires the essential nutrients to maintain good health and uses some compounds found in food to repair itself. Antioxidant-rich foods, such as berries and green leafy veggies can help ward off chronic diseases. This is due to their effects on free radicals. Antioxidants can also have an impact on wrinkles via topically applied essential oils and in the foods we eat. They work by controlling free-radical scavenging activity. In turn, the essential oils may help prevent the damaging effects of everyday ager's and environmental stressors, such as:

- air pollution
- sunlight
- smoke

Anti-Aging Dark Chocolate And Cacao

Eating (or drinking) dark cacao chocolate contains antioxidants that have been shown to help protect the skin against the harmful effects of UV exposure. Cocoa beans have a higher antioxidant capacity than any other food, and 70%+ dark cacao is classified as a superfood because of the high concentration of antioxidant flavanols in cacao helps reduce inflammation of the skin caused by exposure to UV light. Furthermore, eating cacao nibs and dark chocolate can increase circulation in the skin and improve its ability to retain moisture, which can reduce the appearance of wrinkles and help you look years younger. Go ahead! Indulge yourself in this creamy dark pleasure that you'll never have to feel guilty for. Keep in mind this is the pure cacao not milk chocolate as sugar is the primary destroyer of your inner fountain of youth.

Essential Fatty Acids-

Essential fatty acids, such as omega-3 fatty acids, serve important cellular functions. They are a necessary part of the human diet because the body has no biochemical pathway to produce these molecules on its own. Fatty acids have many important functions in the body, including energy storage. If glucose (a type of sugar) isn't available for energy, the body uses fatty acids to fuel the cells instead. Thus a good method of weight loss is to eliminate sugar from the diet.

Food Sources of Essential Fatty Acids:

Fish and other seafood (especially cold-water fatty fish, such as:

- Fish:

    - salmon
    - mackerel
    - tuna
    - herring
    - sardines

- Nuts and seeds:

    - flaxseed
    - chia seeds
    - walnuts

- Plant oils such as:

    - Flaxseed oil
    - Sunflower seed oil

Fish Eggs or Roe Is A Essential Fatty Acid Superfood

If you just like to eat elegant or gourmet food. Nothing tops the list better than Caviar or roe, they are fish eggs.

Caviar is the perfect addition to any diet and is friendly to the following fad diets:

- Paleo
- Keto
- Pescatarian
- Carnivore

Caviar is:

- Has a glycemic index of zero
- High essential fatty acids
- 64% good fat
- Highly carb free
- Sugar free

Fish eggs are filled with quality anti-aging nutrients. One tablespoon of fish roe contains:

- B vitamins
- B12
- Choline
- Magnesium
- Selenium
- Vitamin K2
- Calcium
- Vitamin A
- Zinc
- Iodine
- DHA
- Vitamin D
- and other trace minerals

Drink Hydration

Dehydration is our body's worst aging enemy. Being dehydrated stops our body's ability to flush out toxins. Sip on something hydrating all day long except 30 minutes before each meal, so that you don't neutralize your digestive enzymes or interrupt your alimentary systems natural processes of digestion.

Fountain Of Youth Tea-

- 1 Quart of boiling Water

    - Use spring water or distilled electrolyte water

- 1 Ounce of Earl Grey Tea

    - Green & Black Tea with Bergamot

- Ginger- several slices of organic ginger
- Blueberries (optional)
- Reishi Mushroom pieces (optional)

    - Brew Tea & Let Cool
    - Drop in the ginger while warm

- Chill in fridge overnight
- Enjoy all day

Fountain Of Youth Frozen Smoothie

- 1 Tablespoon - Raw Organic Honey
- 1 Teaspoon Cacao Nibs
- 1 Teaspoon Maca Powder
- ½ Cup Blueberries
- ½ Cup Strawberries
- ½ Cup Cashews, Pecans or Pecans
- ½ Cup Coconut
- 1 cup of ice (made with quality water)

- Pour all ingredients in blender
- Mix and add water or almond milk for consistency
- Enjoy

Fountain Of Youth Infused Water-

- Choose a pure source of spring water,
- Ginger- add slices of fresh ginger,
- Blueberries- fresh or frozen berries
- Lemon or Lime Slices
- Bergamot orange pieces.
- Chill & enjoy.

Recommended Daily Allowance (RDA)

For more information about daily dietary requirements visit the american dietary association website

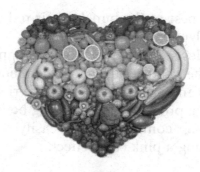

Eat A Rainbow

There are different nutrients in each fruit or vegetable and a variety of phyto-nutrients in the various colors of fruits and vegetables. The list is potentially endless, you can read my other book, "The Balance Diet and Lifestyle" for a breakdown of the health benefits of all of various naturally occurring colors in whole foods but for starters. Apples, for example:

- **Apples**- have over 250 known nutrients and about as many more that we don't even know what they do. An apple a day is said to keep the doctor away. That is because apples are one of the most nutritious foods on the planet. Research shows that eating a daily apple may help reduce the risk of age-related diseases such as:

    o stroke,
    o diabetes,
    o high cholesterol
    o cardiovascular disease.

Apples improve age related conditions such as:

- Eye sight
- Vision
- Immunity/immune system

Apples come in a variety of colors:

    o Red - Red Delicious, Fuji
    o Yellow- Golden Delicious
    o Pink - Pink Lady, Honey Crisp
    o Green- Granny Smith & more

Apple Nutritional Qualities:

- **Red** - apples are the best of the bunch, their red color is from "anthocyanins and heart-healthy polyphenols.
- **Yellow- Yellow apples** start out green but the apple stops making chlorophyll as it matures then the yellow carotenoid pigments mature to golden yellow increasing the sugars and sweetness. These are rich in phytochemicals.
- **Pink**- longest ripening process, longer lasting before falling. The compounds; catechols and phenolic compounds are easily oxidized to terpenoids after contact with air causing a pink color effect.

- **Green** - apples are green because of higher chlorophyll it contains. Green pigments masked by the chlorophyll. Green apples have less sugar and carbs and more fiber, protein, potassium, iron, and vitamin K.

Red Fruits & Veggies

The red pigment in naturally red colored foods are caused by Anthocyanins find these pigments in:

- Apples
- Cranberries
- Pomegranates
- Raspberries
- Beets
- Cherries
- Red cabbage
- Kidney Beans
- Other red or purple foods

Special Nutritional Advice

A good diet is imperative to good health. Balance is the key, eat a balanced diet and read my other book, "The Balanced Diet and Lifestyle"

Exercise Nutrition For Mind & Body Pre-Workout Nutrition Tips:
- Hydrate
- Limit heavy protein
- Eat one to three hours before exercising
- Focus on healthy carbohydrates
- Eat or drink something immediately after exercising
- Combine complex carbohydrates and lean protein

Multi-Vitamin Supplement

If your diet is not what it should be, it's important to take a daily multiple supplement. This is one way to ensure that you are getting a proper nutritional balance of the minimum (RDA) recommended daily allowance of each essential vitamin and mineral which are important for your body to help it maintain good health and proper organ function. Essential nutrients are the fuel our body needs to run smoothly.

If you don't like taking a pill supplement try:

- Low Carb Meal Replacement Bars
- Protein Powders & Shakes
- Weight Loss Shakes
- Eat More Superfoods

    o Avocado
    o Eggs
    o Kale/Spinach/Leafy Greens
    o Seaweed/Algae
    o Nuts, Seeds, Beans & Legumes

Magnesium

Magnesium is one of our body's most used and most important essential minerals and that is why it is also one of the most commonly deficient nutrients more often than all other nutrients because our body uses so much of it. During exercise your muscles need several types of nutrients but it especially uses large quantities of magnesium and without it you get lactic acid build up in the muscle and those agonizing pain wrenching leg cramps, muscle spasms and back pain, PMS and many more dreadful symptoms. It's not just your muscles that rely on magnesium, if you become magnesium deficient you will pretty much feel like a nervous hot mess of a train-wreck. Luckily many foods contain magnesium, such as:

- Dark chocolate
- Spinach
- Bran cereals
- Okra
- Blackeyed Peas
- Almonds
- Peanut Butter

Cacao is a good source of magnesium but unfortunately for chocolate lovers, you can't rely on chocolate alone for magnesium. Your body's cells are a pac-man for magnesium as it is a cofactor in more than 700 enzyme systems that regulate diverse biochemical reactions in the body, including protein synthesis, bone growth, muscle and nerve function, blood glucose control, and blood pressure regulation. Magnesium is required for energy production. In other words, your body functions are pretty much screwed if you don't have enough magnesium because Magnesium is the most important building block for creating a healthy body and maintaining its primary cellular and organ functions as magnesium regulates 700-800 enzyme reactions in the body and of which magnesium is a cofactor. Studies show that eating a diet high in magnesium or by taking a supplement may help reduce symptoms of depression, pain, cramps, stress and anxiety and help relieve many more minor human ailments such as occasional constipation. In fact, you'll know if you're getting enough magnesium as it is also a laxative and if your stool becomes loose then simply cut back on your intake a little regardless your body will eliminate any excess naturally. Some people are better off to get their magnesium naturally through foods they eat instead of taking a supplement such as anyone with kidney failure or other conditions, ask your doctor first.

Stress Age Accelerator

A wide range of studies has shown that the stress caused by things like untreated depression, social isolation, long-term unemployment and anxiety attacks can actually speed-up the aging process by shortening the length of each DNA strand.

Foods For Calming Stress

Dark chocolate researchers have found that, like exercise, dark chocolate may help reduce stress and increase feel good hormones. Experts have long suspected that dark chocolate might help reduce stress and anxiety. A study found that dark chocolate helped reduce perceived stress in students. Other studies have generally found that dark chocolate or cocoa may improve mood as it stimulates the body's endocannabinoid system, yes that's the same system that cannabis stimulates, so yes, a little chocolate can make you feel happier but that doesnt mean go out and get yourself a ton of shitty high-fructose chocolate. Quality matters. Bitter dark cocoa is a rich source of polyphenols, especially flavonoids. Chocolate has a high tryptophan content, tryptophan a calming amino-acid that is also found in turkey that gives us that relaxed feeling after eating thanksgiving turkey. So if you're a vegan or vegetarian chocolate is another way to get a dose of calming tryptophan which the body uses to turn into mood-enhancing neurotransmitters, such as serotonin in the brain. Try to use a daily square of dark chocolate over taking a chill-pill, a daily chocolate habit would be a much better option in the long run because it doesn't block your emotions or leave you feeling like a spaced out airhead all numbed up so that you feel you can't move off the sofa, muchless exercise. Nobody wants to feel like a zombie in the apocalypse. We all want to feel our best and a good quality dark chocolate can help revive a sense of wellbeing in us all. When choosing dark chocolate, aim for 70 percent Cacao or more. Dark chocolate still contains added sugars and fats, so a small serving of 1 to 3 gram square pieces is appropriate and make sure there is no high-fructose syrup or hydrogenated fats in your chocolate.

Turmeric

Turmeric is a spice commonly used in Indian and South-East Asian cooking. The active ingredient in turmeric is called curcumin. Curcumin is as close to a medicine as any food substance as research shows it is anti-inflammatory, anti-bacterial, anti-viral, anti-tumor, and a whole lot of other positive health benefits. Studies show it helps lower anxiety by reducing inflammation and oxidative stress that often increase in people experiencing mood disorders, such as anxiety and depression. Another study found that an increase of curcumin in the diet also increased DHA and reduced anxiety. Turmeric is easy to add to meals. It has minimal flavor, so goes well in smoothies, curries, and casserole dishes. You can also add it to hot milk or nut milk and honey for a delicious drink.

Chamomile

Chamomile is one of the most studied plants and many people around the world use chamomile tea as an herbal remedy because of its immune boosting antibacterial, anti-inflammatory, antioxidant and relaxant properties. Chamomile helps stimulate weight loss and is loaded with calcium, potassium that helps prevent muscle cramps while exercising. It helps detox the body by getting rid of fluid retention. A cup of hot chamomile tea before bedtime may help you get a better night of sleep, also. A recent study found that chamomile did reduce anxiety symptoms. However, it did not prevent new episodes of anxiety. Chamomile tea is useful in calming anxiety. It is readily available and safe to use in high doses.

Vitamin D

Is the sunshine vitamin, it can help improve lack of motivation for exercise. It's important for strong teeth and bones, also it's good for skin and researchers are increasingly linking vitamin D deficiency to mood disorders, such as depression and anxiety. Research proves that vitamin D positively helps improve signs of depression. Other studies on pregnant women and older adults have also highlighted how vitamin D helps improve mood. Vitamin D may also improve seasonal disaffected disorder (SAD) during winter and during prolonged indoor states but whenever you can get out and get some fresh air and sunshine get outside and soak up the vitamin D because the sun stimulates production in your body.

Fermented Foods & Good Bacteria

Yogurt can be either vegan or dairy based. Dairy has tryptophan and vitamin D but offers many other nutrients, too. Yogurt is a good option for everyone as it can be made from fermented rice, soy, coconut kefir or from and fermented milk products, regardless yogurt contains good bacteria, such as *Lactobacillus* and *Bifidobacteria*. There is emerging evidence that these bacteria and fermented products have positive and calming effects on brain health. Yogurt and other dairy products have an anti-inflammatory effect in the body. Some research suggests that chronic inflammation may be partially responsible for anxiety, stress, and depression and therefore fermented foods are a good exercise support food, too.

Studies have found fermented foods help reduce social anxiety, while multiple studies have found that consuming healthful bacteria increases happiness in people. Add yogurt, coconut aminos and other fermented foods to your diet and try some sauerkraut, pickled onions, fermented soy or tofu and kimchi. All can help benefit your natural gut flora which tend to become depleted with age and a poor diet and it may even help reduce your anxiety and stress, too.

Green Tea

For a pre-exercise drink, green tea is the best by far. Green tea contains epigallocatechin gallate (EGCG) is a well-known polyphenol compound is a polyphenol compound concentrated in green tea that may improve mitochondrial function and promote autophagy. Green tea intake has been linked to a reduced risk of all-cause mortality. Green tea also contains an amino acid called theanine, which is a precursor to feel good hormones such as serotonin and dopamine L- theanine elevates levels of GABA, as well as increases serotonin and dopamine levels. It helps with motivation and additionally, L- theanine helps to lower levels of corticosterone stress hormone. As with many natural foods and plants that have incredible health benefits, Green tea is receiving increased scrutiny by those who try to discredit it because they can't profit from its use. The fact is, green tea compounds have a real science-backed effect on mood disorders. Theanine has anti-anxiety and calming effects on the brain chemistry and additionally it offers a natural mild boost of caffeine which can give you a quick energy pick-up, also. Green tea is easy to add to your daily diet. It is a healthier replacement for soft drinks and alcoholic beverages. A human research trial, found that 200 mg of theanine improved self-reported relaxation, increased calmness and reduced tension.

Some Natural Sources of Theanine are:

- Coffee

- Tea
- Guarana
- Yerba Mate
- Mushrooms

Post Exercise Recovery

Athletic people need extra nutrition. It is important to eat a balanced diet. If you are having problems with meal planning, seek individualized nutritional advice from a professionally trained nutritionist. Additionally, water and hydration is important when we exercise, as exercise makes us perspire and can become dehydrated. Replenish electrolytes after exercise we often sweat. The more you sweat the more nutrients you lose and the greater your risk of developing a nutritional deficiency. The more you work your muscles the more nutrition your body needs to prevent the body from pulling nutrients from the organ systems and nutrient reserves. Everyone needs a proper balance of essential nutrients and should follow a balanced diet according to their daily recommended nutritional requirements. We use our muscles when we exercise. Just two pounds of muscle can burn ten pounds of fat in a year. Therefore, we need muscle fuel for the extra work our muscles do during exercise. Muscle is protein just as meat and flesh is protein.

One of the best foods for an athlete is protein. Protein should be increased in body-building and training diets and proteins are excellent for energy. The enzymes protease and peptidase are needed to properly digest protein. Caution should be used to increase the protein intake to balance your sources of proteins without adding animal sources. Therefore, vegetable proteins such as soy, beans, nuts, whole grains and fish are the best choices. Red meat proteins such as beef produce acid ash residues which in excess, contribute to unhealthy acid imbalances in the body, and therefore, should be eaten only in moderation. Chicken, Turkey and Fish are better meat choices but still produce acid residues.

Anti-Aging Nutrition

Type 1 & II Collagen protein is important for anti-aging benefits. Extra proteins are necessary for athletes and muscle building benefits; however, a person can eat too much protein, a high meat, high acid diet may result in high urea and heavy uric acid concentrations have been linked to deaths in active athletes. Athletes need minerals and amino acids. Mineral deficiencies can lead to strokes in athletes. We sweat out a lot of trace nutrients during intense exercise. That is why I believe it's not healthy to over do exercise, either. Moderation is key. Replenishing essential nutrients is important for the body to maintain good health and proper function. Too much protein is unhealthy and can lead to a buildup of excess urea & acid residues that cause heart stress if the protein is not digested properly. The body needs enzymes from raw plants to digest protein. Urea's are the undigested proteins within the body. A sign of high urea in the body are unusual or pronounced deep wrinkles in the forehead area another symptom is feeling fatigued when you wake up in the morning. With all the high protein training food supplements on the market one must be aware of these warning signs to reduce risk of toxic urea levels. If you suspect you may have this problem, consult with your doctor. High protein shakes and food supplements should be used with caution to keep a healthy balance of nutrition by including other healthy foods in your diet. Periodically, one should give the body a rest from the hard digestion of high protein food supplements and allow the body adequate intervals of alkalizing foods and short fast to stimulate autophagy and to offset any imbalance that may be occurring within the body.

Protein Muscle Power

Protein provides branched chain amino acids for sustained endurance. The "Critical Cluster" branched chain amino acids are used as a powerful source of energy during exercise. The "Critical Cluster" branched chain amino acids are Valine, Arginine, Leucine, Isoleucine, and Glutamine. Protein helps stimulate the release of the anabolic hormones that will promote new muscle formation during exercise and result in an increase in lean body mass and a decrease in fat mass. Arginine plays a major role in stimulating the release of anabolic hormones that promote healthy muscle definition and formation. Arginine can be made by the body from ornithine and is done in maintaining good health and homeostasis. Arginine speeds wound healing and has immunity enhancing benefits. Arginine helps the body best when in a stressed state. Arginine may be used for better muscle formation, reduction of physical stress, and in for developing a strong and healthy immune system. Numerous studies in Olympic athletes have shown the positive effects of supplemental Arginine. Protein helps increase your ability to utilize oxygen, thus helping you sustain high-intensity exercise for a longer period. If you weight training more protein is required to have a protein shake and for up to date information on nutrition visit the American Dietetics Association website.

Oxidative Stress & Age Related Physical Frailty

Frailty is an important health problem for older adults. Its clinical significance is increasingly being demonstrated and recognized. The pathogenesis of frailty involves:

- insulin resistance
- inflammation
- sarcopenia
- adiposity
- age-related hormone decline
- nervous system dysfunction.

What remains unclear is how these abnormalities of multiple physiologic systems occur as we age. The answer may lie in the increased oxidative stress that occurs during aging. Correlative human studies using different markers of oxidative stress consistently showed that increased oxidative stress independently predicts frailty.

Transgenic mice with high oxidative stress display pathologies and phenotypes resembling those of frailty.

Oxidative stress can cause frailty by the following cellular mechanisms:

- mitochondrial dysfunction;
- damage to proteins critical for maintaining homeostasis and muscle function;
- endoplasmic reticulum (ER) stress;
- cellular apoptosis;
- cellular senescence; and
- abnormal cellular signaling.

Oxidative stress and its downstream cellular pathogenic pathways may offer the targets for prevention and intervention strategies against frailty.

Bitters

Bitter flavors are not typically sought for in the typical western diet. Americans tend to prefer sweet or rich flavors. Nutritional bitters are an anti-aging food source with many valuable anti-aging qualities and benefits that have been used since the beginning of time and they are important in maintaining good health and proper digestion as well as enhancing organ function. The following are a few safe common bitter herbs:

- Oregon grape
- Chamomile
- Gentian
- Wormwood

- Chicory
- Neem
- Hops
- Goldenseal
- Angelica
- Horehound
- Centaury
- Mugwort
- Bitter melon
- Ginger root
- Bergamot
- Grapefruit
- Lemons
- Limes
- Wild lettuce
- Milk thistle
- Horseradish
- Artichoke
- Aloe vera
- Yarrow
- Myrrh
- Dandelion
- Boneset
- Tea
- Turnip Greens
- Radishes

Additionally, these bitter herbs, spices and foods gently detoxify your body and are safe to be consumed on a daily basis to stimulate your digestive juices and so you get the most out of the nutrition these plants offer to help your body rid itself of toxins, inflammation and mucus catterah.

Diosmin

Diosmin is a flavone glycoside which is found in a natural structure in the pericarps of different citrus fruits flavone glycoside is obtained by dehydrogenation of hesperidin. Diosmin was first isolated from Figwort. Clinical evidence suggests that diosmin is a safe, nontoxic compound that is successfully used to treat:

- spider veins,

- varicose veins,
- chronic venous disease,
- hemorrhoids and
- diabetes

Diosmin has been used for over a decade in Europe. It activates the enzymes of carbohydrate metabolism and is found to reverse the abnormalities.

Diosmin alleviates:

- Oxidative stress of the liver, and kidneys and
- Helps restore elevated blood glucose and
- Restores lipid profiles to normal.

Hence, diosmin has been shown to improve factors associated with diabetic complications.

Your Inner Cannabinoid System

The Endocannabinoid System(ECS) is a molecular system within the body that is responsible for regulating and balancing many processes in the body, including:

- immune response
- communication between cells
- appetite and metabolism
- memory
- and many more

The endocannabinoid system is comprised of the following:

- endocannabinoids
- enzymes that regulate ECS synthesis
- enzymes that regulate ECS degradation
- prototypical cannabinoid receptors (CB1 and CB2)
- some non-cannabinoid receptors, and
- an uncharacterised ECS transport system.

Endocannabinoids are produced naturally by cells in the human body. These endocannabinoids are made from fat-like molecules within cell membranes and are synthesized on-demand. THC and marajuana contain cannabinoids but a better source is hemp without the psychoactive compound of THC.

Hemp DNA Health Benefits

DNA can be damaged and it can also be repaired. DNA (deoxyribonucleic acid) is the hereditary material found in humans, animals, and organisms. DNA is in every cell of your body. The nucleus of each cell contains DNA, which contain structures that are our 23 pairs of chromosomes. One thing that we now know that repairs DNA is Hemp.

Hemp Protein Repairing Smoothie

1 Scoop of Hemp protein powder
1 Cup Spinach
¼ Cup Blueberries (frozen)
¼ Banana (frozen)
¼ Turmeric Tea (ground turmeric, cinnamon, ginger)
1 cup Almond Milk
¼ cup Ice
1 cup water

Optional Additions:

- Your favorite protein powder brand,
- Enzymes,
- NMN,
- Carnosine,
- Fiestin powder or
- Any of your favorite anti-aging liquids or supplements.

Blend all ingredients in a blender, garnish with:

- lemon or
- mint,
- fresh slices of strawberries
- Cinnamon sticks or sprinkle of cinnamon.

Drink-up, enjoy, power-up!

Aging & Genes

Genes contain information needed to manufacture functional molecules called proteins and also a few other genes produce molecules to help cells assemble proteins. The journey from gene to protein is complex and controlled in each cell. It consists of two major steps:

1. transcription and
2. translation

Together, transcription and translation are known as:

• gene expression

During the process of transcription, information that is stored in a gene' s DNA is then transferred into a similar molecule called RNA (ribonucleic acid) in the cell nucleus.

RNA and DNA are both made up of a chain of nucleotide bases, but they have slightly different chemical properties. The type of RNA that contains the information for making a protein is called "messenger RNA" (mRNA) because it carries the information, or message, from the DNA out of the nucleus into the cell's cytoplasm into the gene's direct protein production.

For instance, a protein is a long chain of amino acids that can also act as an enzyme that can trigger specific chemical reactions within the body. One function of proteins is to boost the body's immune system.

There are many factors that cause damaged DNA:

• Oxidation,
• UV Radiation from the sun,
• Radiation from X Rays,
• Viruses,
• Mycotoxins
• Plant toxins, and
• Man-made chemicals:

    ○ Herbicides
    ○ Pesticides
    ○ Chlorine,

- Hydrocarbons,
- Smoke,
- Pollution and more.

Some results of damaged DNA are:

- Premature aging in skin
- Hair and Nail Loss,
- Cancer,
- Diabetes
- Mellitus
- Diabetes
- Parkinsons,
- Alzheimers,
- Chronic fatigue syndrome,
- Weight gain
- Inflammation
- Neurological damage
- Nerve Damage
- and many other conditions.

Your cells cannot function properly if your DNA is damaged. However, the cells can reverse the damage themselves through chemical processes.

Simple Solution For DNA Repair

Hemp seed and hemp seed oil have been found to be a factor in DNA repair.

Nutritionally, hemp contains essential fatty acids needed by the human body and Omega 3 is the essential for cellular repair including skin cells. Hemp offers the perfect ratio for optimum human health benefits as follows:

- 3:1 ratio of Omega fatty acids
- Omega 3
- Omega 6
- Hemp is 65% protein

  - 35% of Hemp is edestin:
  - globulin edestin protein

Edestin Protein

Protein is a major factor in DNA repair as the cells use protein to correct the DNA damage.

- Edestin protein is found only in hemp seed.
- Edestin aids digestion and is relatively phosphorus free.
- Edestin protein is similar to the human body's own globular proteins found in blood plasma.
- Edestin protein produces antibodies which are vital to maintain a healthy immune system.

Since edestin protein closely resembles the globulin in blood plasma, it's compatible with the human digestive system. This may be the reason why there are no reported food allergies to hemp foods. Hemp protein contain:

- Edestin protein is easily digestible by the body.
- Edestin protein contains glutamic acid.

Glutamic acid is a stress fighting neurotransmitter that helps people deal with mental stress.

Albumin protein

Hemp also contains Albumin protein.

- Albumin is similar to the protein found in egg whites.
- Albumin is the current industry standard for protein supplement evaluation.
- Albumin is a high quality globulin protein
- Albumin protein is highly digestible
- Albumin is a major source of free radical scavengers.
- Albumin helps repair DNA

Digestion transforms hemp protein into amino acids which are the basic building blocks required for the growth and maintenance of bodily tissue.

Hemp protein contains:
- All 20 amino acids
- 9 essential amino acids (EAAs).

The essential amino acids are labeled "essential" because the human body cannot produce them on its own. A diet that is deficient of EAAs may lead to degenerative conditions such as:

- Dementia
- Decreased immunity,
- Digestive problems,
- Depression,
- Fertility issues,
- Lower mental alertness,
- Slowed growth in children,
- Slow wound healing
- and many other health issues.

Hemp Vrs. Soy Protein

Hemp is second only to soy in protein content, but when hemp protein is compared to soy protein it should be noted that hemp does not contain trypsin inhibitors that soy does. Trypsin is an enzyme that is essential to nutrition. Since hemp protein is free of the tyrosine inhibitors that are normally found in soy protein, hemp is one of the best plant protein sources and since hemp is the highest source of Edestin protein, which is responsible for boosting the immune system and because it can help repair DNA damage, it is a perfect addition to your longevity diet.

Your body produces its own protein waste in the form of dead cells.

Protein The Tissue Transformers:

All flesh and meat is protein, including our own bodies. Everyday your body needs to replace more than 6-10 ounces of protein but the average person consumes only 2.5 ounces of protein a day. Some studies show that even if you are a vegetarian, your body still has the same amount of protein and carbohydrates as if you were an animal protein eater because when you eat too much protein or meat, it interferes with the body's self-cleaning mechanisms of eliminating old cell debris protein waste.

Chapter 13

Autophagy: Your Body's Automatic Self-Cleaning System

The body's internal self-cleaning process is called "Autophagy" and through this process your body can use its own protein from damaged or dead cells and bacteria.

"Out With The Old And In With The New"

Just as your dead skin cells shed daily or you can slough off with exfoliation, the internal tissues die off and regenerate on their own, too. We can boost the renewal processes by assisting our internal Autophagy mechanisms.

- **Autophagy**- the body's ability to self-eat its own protein garbage waste.
- **Keratin**- epidermis hair skin and nails.
- **Lysosomes**- your body can decompose dead cell debris protein into amino acids.

Autophagy is the body's internal self-cleaning mechanism.

Fasting Triggers Autopahagy

Fasting is the quickest way to achieve a state of Autophagy in the body and induce your internal cells into self-cleaning mode. However, those individuals who are very toxic may become ill from releasing too many toxins at once during an autophagy detox. Rapid detox can cause unpleasant symptoms such as:

- Hunger pangs
- Nausea
- Vomiting
- Irritability
- Headaches

These unpleasant symptoms are why it is recommended for beginners to seek medical clearance first or start out with mini-fast or intermittent fasting. Then after your body becomes accustomed to fasting you can go longer on a fast and try water fasting.

Autophagy Fasting Exercise

Autophagy is the body's internal self-cleaning system. The meaning of the word Autophagy is "Auto" means self and "phagy" means eat. Autophagy is the word for "self-eating or a better way to look at it is to fast or do exercises or treatments to trigger and activate our body's own internal self cleaning. During fasting, the process of autophagy initiates after 18-20 hours of fasting, with the maximal benefits occurring after depriving yourself of solid food 48–72 hours, which sounds like misery, but Autophagy can be triggered by staying a little bit cold and hungry and by doing short burst high intensity exercise or by consuming miniscule portions of certain food substances such as copious amounts of bergamot tea on an otherwise empty stomach.

Autophagy & Skin Cell Renewal

When we fast it jump-starts our body's Autophagy. Autophagy is a physiological means in which the body eats what is not working effectively within itself to liberate energy for new cells to work in an optimal state. Autophagy was first observed in 1962 by Keith R. Porter and his student Thomas Ashford at the Rockefeller Institute, in 1974. In the 1990s several groups of scientists independently discovered autophagy-related genes. Notably, Yoshinori Ohsumi and Michael Thumm examined starvation-induced non-selective autophagy. Dr. Ohsumi later won the Nobel prize for his research discoveries in 2016.

Autophagosomes

Part of your body's self cleaning mechanisms are Autophagosomes, they are double-membraned vesicles that contain cellular material slated to be degraded by autophagy, your body's internal self cleaning mechanism. Your glucagon level is the one that initiates autophagy. "When your body is low on sugar through fasting or ketosis, it brings the positive stress that wakes up the survival repairing mode.

3 Types of Autophagy

(AMPK) 5' adenosine monophosphate-activated protein kinase is an enzyme that plays a role in cellular energy homeostasis, largely to activate glucose and fatty acid uptake and oxidation when cellular energy is low. AMPK activates when your fasting

Working Out- activates when you do short burst high-intensity.

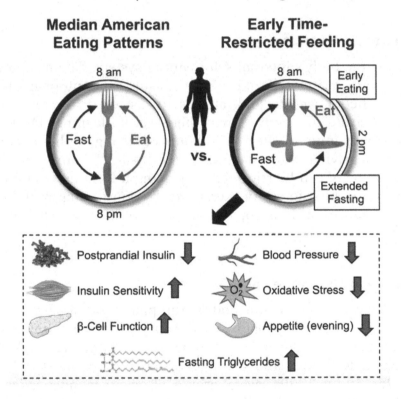

Autophagy Stimulating Foods-

- Green Tea- EGCG stimulates and increases autophagy in the liver, the autophagic flux.
- Ginger-6-Shogaol induces autophagic cell death.
- Curcumin- Turmeric activates the phosphorylation of AMPK and autophagy

- Reishi Mushroom- has autophagic effects and suppresses the proliferation of cancer cells suppresses the phosphorylation of mitogen-activated protein kinase (p38 MAPK) while activating autophagy.

Autophagy Without Fasting

- Nicotinamide Mononucleotide (NMN)- Nicotinamide mononucleotide is a nucleotide derived from ribose and nicotinamide. NMN is made from B vitamins in the body, and is a molecule naturally occurring in all life forms.
- Dopamine- Derived from citrus in the Rutaceae plant family, commonly known as the rue or citrus family, of flowering plants, usually placed in the order Sapindales. Species of the family generally have flowers that divide into four or five parts, usually with strong scents. They range in form and size from herbs to shrubs and large trees.

Autophagy & Exercise

Recent studies suggest that exercise stimulates autophagy in both muscles and other bodily tissues. Autophagy is our body's own internal self-cleaning mechanism. It's the process that the body eats up all the dead cells to make way for new ones to regenerate and it's important because nobody needs a bunch of dead waste sticking around. Additionally, muscle-derived myokines after exercise help induce autophagy in liver cells.

- The best exercise to stimulate autophagy is by doing a mix of:

  - resistance training and
  - short-burst high-intensity interval training
  - cardio

- Too much exercise negates some autophagy benefits.

  - only do high intensity exercise only about 30 minutes per day.
  - high intensity exercise is a stressor of the body and mind.
  - it's unnatural to deliberately push yourself into a physical state beyond your capacity and it can cause harm
  - The hippocratic oath to good health care is "first of all do no harm".
  - Exercising yourself beyond your means is an equivalent to being in combat and that is too stressful and damaging to the body.

o healthy exercise should be uncomfortable but it should never be painful and

o exercise doesn't have as much anti-aging benefit by pushing your pain threshold or by prolonging a high-intensity state of stress on the body is counter productive and accelerates aging of the joints and musculoskeletal system.

Autophagy Alternatives

Autophagy is automatically stimulated during a fast. However, many people can't fast due to various reasons, low blood sugar or self-control issues. In those cases, there is an alternative approach. Our body goes into autophagy automatically when we feel a little bit hungry or a little bit cold. So in that sense it's always good to feel a little bit cold and hungry.

- Do intermittent fasting for 18 hours overnight through till midday. 7 pm till 12 noon or 8pm-1pm.
- Apply an ice pack to the upper back/in neck area to trigger self-healing mechanisms in the body.
- Sip water or unsweetened tea during your fast.

Anti-Aging Autophagy

Autophagy is important for Anti-Aging. Our society is all about satiation but staying satiated is overindulgent and can block our autophagy. Some foods that stimulate autophagy are:

- Cinnamon
- Ginseng
- Garlic
- Chaga
- Reishi Mushrooms
- Pomegranate
- Elderberries
- Bergamot
- Berberine
- Resveratrol
- Coffee
- Green tea
- Turmeric

- Ginger

Ultimate Anti Aging Longevity Smoothie

2 Cups Spring Water Ice (use portable ice maker)
1 Cup Frozen Strawberries & Blueberries
¼ Cup Hemp Protein Powder
1 T Collagen Protein Powder
½ Cup Coconut
¼ Cup Tofu
¼ Cup Cilantro
¼ Cup Kale
¼ Cup Spinach
½ Cup Broccoli
½ T Pine Pollen
¼ T Ginger
¼ T NMN powder
¼ T Carnosine powder
1 T Marine Algae
1 T Tumeric Tea
1 T Bergamot Tea

Liposomal Smoothie Additions:

1 T Resveratrol
¼ T NAD
¼ T Soursop

Blend all ingredients in a blender.
Garnish with fresh fruit and herbs.
Enjoy!

Exercise Triggers Glucagon Induced Atophagy

Always keep in mind that in the first 20 minutes of moderate to intense exercise performance, muscle glycogen is used as the primary energy source and provides glucose for muscle fueling. By exercising until your oxygen reserves it will cause your body to use protein out of the muscle to cause a new formation of glucose this is called gluconeogenesis. It is important to exercise longer than 20 minutes to get into the most efficient fat burning phase of exercise. After this initial 20-minute phase of exercise, fatty acids and the branched chain amino acids are the muscle's major energy source. Drink water after exercise and do not eat sugary substances immediately after exercise until the hormones decline or you will crash after your workout because the liver will secrete these hormones.

When you exercise, the body produces hormones that block insulin so your body can effectively use the glucose from your muscles and from the bloodstream. One of the best foods for athletes is protein. Protein should be increased in diets of training athletes. Protein is excellent for increasing energy levels in athletes. The enzymes protease and peptidase are needed to properly digest protein. Caution should be used to increase the protein intake without adding animal sources. Therefore, vegetable proteins such as soy, beans, nuts, whole grains and fish are the best choices. Proteins such as beef & chicken produce acid ash residues which in excess, contribute to unhealthy acid imbalances in the body, and therefore, should be eaten only in moderation. Extra proteins are necessary for athletes however, high urea and heavy uric acid concentrations have been linked to deaths in active athletes. Urea's are the undigested proteins within the body. A sign of high urea in the body are unusual or pronounced deep wrinkles in the forehead area another symptom is feeling fatigued when you wake up in the morning. With all the high protein training food supplements on the market one must be aware of these warning signs to reduce risk of toxic urea levels. Periodically, one should give the body a rest from the hard digestion of these high protein food supplements and allow the body adequate intervals of alkalizing to offset any imbalance that may be occurring within the body.

Example Autophagy Menu & Regimen:

Autophagy is triggered by hunger so after a night's sleep is a good time to periodically allow your body to go into a state of autophagy and allow the body to do its internal self-cleaning. An easy way is to skip breakfast and have a late lunch, drinking only fluids that stimulate autophagy and then breaking the fast with a fresh veggie juice, whole raw fruit, protein shake or a salad. Drink a glass of water 30 minutes before or 30 minutes after eating. You may add lemon cucumber, mint or grapefruit slices to your water.

Morning

- Drink 1 Glass of water
- Drink 1 Cup of black coffee or
- Drink 1 Cup of green tea,
- Drink 1 Cup of earl grey tea or pea flower tea

Late Lunch (after noon)

- Collagen Protein Shake or
- Small salad

  - 1 cup of arugula leaves
  - ½ lemon squeezed over leaves
  - 1 Tablespoon Berries as topper
  - 1 Tablespoon of raw seeds or nuts as topper
  - 1 Tablespoon of Parmesan cheese
  - 1 glass of water

Afternoon Snack

- ½ Avocado (large or whole small) or
- ½ Grapefruit or
- ½ Cup of yogurt (low-fat dairy or non dairy)
- 1oz. dark chocolate (try Anti-Aging Brand)
- 1 Glass of water
- 1 Cup of Detox Tea (try Anti-Aging Brand)

Dinner

- 2 cups- Steamed Asparagus, Broccoli or Raw Salad
- 1 Cup Quinoa or Brown rice or boiled potatoes
- 1 T. coconut aminos (poured over the rice)
- 3 oz of fish or lean meat or meat alternative
- 1 glass of water
- 1 T. Rice Vinegar or Sweet Balsamic (veggie topper)

Snack

- 1 Apple or orange (or 1-cup other whole fruit)
- 6 Almonds
- 4 Olives
- 1 Glass of water

Bed Time (optional 2 hours before sleeping fast)

- Cup of camomile tea or other night time herb tea blend
- **Your choice of only one of the following:**

- o 1 Celery stick with 1 teaspoon nut butter
- o 1 Carrot
- o 5-8 Almonds
- o 1 Tangerine, Date or Fig
- o 1 T. Roe

Bed Time (best option for Autophagy fast)

- 1- Glass of water or 3 oz. cup of
- 1- Night Time relaxing herbal tea (caffeine free)

The goal is to achieve autophagy, and that can be done with intermittent fasting.

- **Intermittent Fasting**- is staying a little hungry at all times for several days. This is good for triggering autophagy.

  - o Not eating for 3 hours before bed & then you fast while you sleep.
  - o Not eating until noon, thereafter, hydrate in the mornings.

    - ▪ Drinking infused water instead of eating in between meals (citrus bergamot)
    - ▪ Drinking tea- polyphenols 3 - 6 cups day

Breaking The Intermittent Fast-

  - ▪ An apple a day keeps the doctor away
  - ▪ 1 cup of brown rice or quinoa
  - ▪ Protein cycle (confuse the metabolism)
  - ▪ On a low protein day 5-10% of calories (a veggie day)
  - ▪ On a high protein day is 45% protein (keto)
  - ▪ On a good fat day- nuts, eggs, good fats
  - ▪ **Diet** - There is no one size fits all diet.
  - ▪ Low or no processed carbs -
  - ▪ 1 whole bread daily or make it a whole meal.

Fasting Autophagy By Meal Timing

Your meal timing can trigger autophagy without making fasting too difficult. Fasting overnight and waiting till noon can make a difference in our body without feeling like you're starving yourself to death. An in-depth review of the science of recently published in New England Journal of Medicine sheds some light. Fasting is evolutionarily embedded within our physiology, triggering several essential cellular functions. Flipping the switch from a fed to fasting state does more than help us burn calories and lose weight. The researchers combed through dozens of animal and human studies to explain how simple fasting improves metabolism, lowering blood sugar; lessens inflammation and improves a range of other health issues from arthritic pain to asthma; and even triggers autophagy to help clear out toxins and damaged cells, lowering the risk of cancer and enhances brain function thus lowering the risk of age related brain decline disorders such as alzhimers and dementia.

Circadian Rhythm During Fasting

Research has provided evidence to suggest that the circadian rhythm during fasting in which meals are restricted to an 8-10 hour period of the daytime, is effective, but each individual person will need to use an eating approach that works for them and is sustainable to their needs.

When Intermittent Fasting Is Not Ok

People with advanced diabetes or who are on medications for diabetes, people with a history of eating disorders like anorexia and bulimia, and pregnant or breastfeeding women should not attempt intermittent fasting unless under the close supervision of a physician who can monitor them.

4 ways to use Intermittent Fasting for better health

1. Avoid sugars and refined grains. Instead, eat fruits, vegetables, beans, lentils, whole grains, lean proteins, and healthy fats (a sensible, plant-based, Mediterranean-style diet).
2. Let your body burn fat between meals. Don't snack. Be active throughout your day. Build muscle tone.
3. Consider a simple form of intermittent fasting. Limit the hours of the day when you eat, and for best effect, make it earlier in the day (between 7 am to 3 pm, or even 10 am to 6 pm, but definitely not in the evening before bed).
4. Avoid snacking or eating at nighttime, all the time

Chapter 14

Super Supplements That Activate Your Fountain Of Youth

Anti-Aging Supplements

Today, it is possible to find almost any form of supplements, be it enzymes, hormones, vitamins or minerals. Supplements for various health and beauty purposes are readily available, and so are those that aid in reducing the signs of aging.

While it is always better to opt for natural methods through improving diet, supplements can speed up the journey to looking more youthful. Supplements, when taken with care and precaution can be very beneficial in attaining numerous health benefits. Some of the more well-known supplements available for aging issues include the following options:

- **Antioxidants**
  "Antioxidant" is definitely a buzzword when it comes to healthy food, but what exactly does it mean? Antioxidants are substances that protect our bodies against free radicals — unstable molecules that are produced when our bodies break down food, or by exposure to pollution and radiation. Free radicals can damage our body's healthy cells, and are thought to play a part in the onset of certain diseases, including Alzheimer's, cancer and heart disease.

- **Anti-Aging Proteins**
  One of the reasons we begin to show signs of aging is because it becomes harder for proteins into the cells.
  The youthful appearance and the condition of your hair, skin, and nails depends on three proteins, known as your "3 Beauty Proteins" and they are:

1. **Collagen**

    Collagen "plumps" your skin from the inside out. It removes fine lines and wrinkles, and prevents them from forming. In addition, collagen is essential for strong, healthy bones and joints. Microminerals "turn on" the collagen-generating cells in your body known as fibroblasts.

2. **Elastin**

    Elastin gives your skin its ability to stretch and elasticity to maintain its shape while it helps prevent fine lines and wrinkles from developing. Elastin is also vital to the proper functioning of the organs and eyes.

3. **Keratin**

    Keratin is the protein that's packed into your hair shaft. It gives your hair thickness, body, strength, and elasticity. Plus, keratin gives your nails strength and clarity. Studies suggest the fact that microminerals stimulate the keratin-producing cells in your body known as keratinocytes.

1. **Collagen-**

    Collagen declines in our 20's and follows the decline in estrogen levels and testosterone levels. There is a big dip in collagen in your late 40's. It is important for the health of our dermis to consume 20 grams of collagen daily. Taking a collagen supplement is a good way to start your anti-aging diet. Important points to remember about dietary collagen.

- There are 20+ types of dietary collagen
- It's important to get multi forms of collagen
- Bone broth is a good source of collagen.
- Grass fed bovine clean sourced
- Use high quality sources to avoid contamination.

Collagen offers the following health improvements:

- Strength-

    o Strong muscles,
    o Healthy joints &
    o Connective tissues

- Skeletal health-

- Spine
- Structural health
- Joints
- Joint health and
- Connective tissue health

- Beauty-

  - healthy skin
  - Healthy hair
  - healthy nails

Collagen Benefits On Skin

Collagen is a complex protein that is naturally produced by the body and consists of 19 amino acids. Collagen has different types, but the one found in your skin is type

- Collagen makes your skin:

  - Stronger
  - Thicker
  - Less prone to damage
  - Decreases risk of disease
  - Helps keep the skin hydrated
  - Reduces wrinkles
  - Freckles
  - Scars.

New scientific research shows that ingesting a collagen supplement is of great benefit to the body so remember to take a daily collagen supplement.

- Collagen also helps:

  - protect nerves
  - Protect the aging brain

2. **Elastin:**
   Your skin's ability to spring back after stretching it is known as elasticity. Skin naturally loses some of its ability to stretch and bounce back with aging. There are many treatments for improving skin elasticity but in order for them to work

successfully we must be healthy from within. If you notice a rapid decline in your skin's health, it's time to access your diet or toxin exposures to recognize if there may be a systemic factor at play. Some environmental factors can accelerate the accumulation of progerin and speed up the aging process. such as:

- Smoking or
- Mold illness/Mycotoxins
- Sun exposure and
- Bad skin-care habits,
- Alcohol consumption
- Sugar consumption

Look for what is hidden that may be damaging your skin and cause a loss of elasticity. Your skin elasticity can be improved with Lifestyle changes, such as:

- Exercise
- Wearing sunscreen,
- Drinking more water
- Avoid exposure to mold mycotoxins (DNA damage)

These are only a few lifestyle tips that can help improve elasticity and slow down and minimize aging effects. Increasing your intake of water can help as water makes it easier for healthy skin to spring back to the surface. Exercise can also boost elastin, increase blood flow and nutrition to the skin, enhance elastin production and help firm your skin surface.

3. **Keratin Protein**- Keratin is a type of structural protein found in your hair, skin, and nails but humans cannot digest hair because we don't have the enzymes that are needed to digest keratin from hair and some supplement companies use hair and feathers in their oral keratin supplements, which is not a good idea. The best way to boost your body's keratin production is by eating the following foods that promote keratin production in your body, unless you are allergic to any of the foods then obviously its is not recommended but for the rest of us try these foods to improve keratin production:

- Protein sources
- Eggs
- Onions
- Salmon
- Sweet potatoes

- Sunflower seeds
- Mangoes
- Garlic
- Kale

Best Anti-Aging Supplements

Like superfoods, there are also specific supplements that are considered super supplements. The following are some of those super anti-aging substances:

Cycloastragenol-

CA-98's (CA) protects against the issues associated with aging at their root and is known to support a great number of beneficial health effects. It is an extract from Astragalus. It helps to improve:

- the human immune system.
- helps in regulating the respiratory system.

Many food supplements are from Astragalus root extracts. One of such product is CA-98

- CA-98 helps Telomere / DNA health
- Naturally supports telomere length repair
- Increases energy levels,
- Builds muscles, and
- Improve mood.
- Support your body's ability to aid DNA repair to lengthen telomeres.
- Supports cell replication
- aids immune function and
- Improves overall wellbeing.
- Use to naturally protect and restore your cellular health!

Healthy DNA and longer telomeres are key to longevity and better overall health. The health of your skin, hair, nails, and body systems are all dependent on your body's ability to heal and generate new cells.

Dr. Joy's Ultimate 11 Age-Support Supplements:

- **1. Chemistry Balancer**

  - Adaptogens
  - Trace Minerals
  - Calcium
  - Magnesium

- **2. Hormone Balancer**

  - DIM
  - DHEA
  - Pine Pollen

- **3. Essential Nutrients**

  - Multi-Vitamin
  - Multi-Mineral
  - Trace Minerals

- **4. Brain Support Anti Oxidants**

  - Ginkgo
  - Vinpocetine
  - Proanthocyanidins

    - Pycnogenol
    - Pine Bark

- **5. Anti-Inflammatory**

  - Curcumin
  - Quercetin
  - Boswellia
  - Co-Q10

- **6. Detoxifier-**

  - SOD/Superoxide Dismutase
  - Detox Tea

- Green Tea
- Earl Grey/ Bergamot Tea

- **7. Autophagy Stimulators-**

  - Fisitin,
  - Bergamot,
  - NMN

- **8. DNA Gene Support-**

  - NMN
  - NAD+
  - Resveratrol

- **9. Structural Support-**

  - Skin
  - Hair
  - Nails
  - Joints

    - Collagen
    - Hyaluronic Acid
    - Glucosamine
    - Chondroitin
    - Bioflavonoids

- **10. Enzymes**

  - Digestive enzymes
  - Systemic enzymes
  - Proteolytic enzymes
  - ATP
  - AMPK

- **11. Immune Boosters**

  - Probiotics
  - Beta Glucans
  - Prebiotics

    ○ Colostrum

Solution For Taking Too Many Pills

If taking 11 supplements a day is too much, you could take 5 one day and 6 the next or rotate these 11 supplements out and take them every other day. Consuming these 11 daily is ideal but consuming them at least 3-5 days a week is better than not taking them at all and our body needs these compounds to help maintain its function over the years as you age. The other option is that you can get some of them from the foods you eat and drink.

Fisetin Super Anti-Age

Fisetin helps delay the development and the onset of aging phenotypes, attenuate severity of age-related diseases, improve resiliency, and enhances longevity. Fisetin can be extracted from fruits and herbal sources. It can be found in juices, wines and teas. It can be found in many plants as it is a coloring agent in plants. It is also found in many fruits and vegetables, such as:

- Strawberries
- Apples
- Persimmons
- Onions
- Cucumbers

Fisetin Neutralizes Progerin, The Bad Skin Wrinkling Protein

Progerin "The Bad Protein"

Progerin is the bad protein that causes wrinkling and the appearance of aging. In 2007 researchers at the National Institute of Health discovered that progerin was also present in the normal skin and fat cells of healthy people and, most significantly, progentin increases with age by about 3% each year as well as do wrinkles occur with the increase of the "bad protein".

Ultimate Anti-Aging DNA Repairing Smoothie

2 Cups Ice (Spring Water Ice made with portable ice maker)
¼ Cup Hemp Protein Powder
1 T Collagen Protein Powder
1 Cup Your Choice:
- Frozen Pineapple, Strawberries or Blueberries

¼ Cup Your Choice:
- Broccoli, Bok Choy, Cauliflower or Cabbage

¼ Cup Your Choice:
- Arugula, Kale or Spinach

¼ Cup Your Choice:
- Tofu, Tempeh or Miso paste

¼ Cup Coconut
½ T Pine Pollen
¼ T Ginger
¼ T NMN powder
¼ T Carnosine powder
1 T Marine Algae
1 T Tumeric Tea
1 T Bergamot Tea

Liposomal Additions:

1 T Resveratrol, ¼ T NAD or ¼ T Soursop

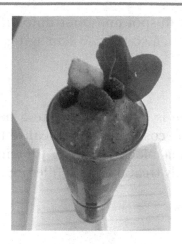

What Happens With Protein With Age

As we age optimal protein utilization declines. At the same time, our cells also become less able to remove the bad protein. In turn, the accumulation of a bad protein, progerin begins to reduce the skin cells' ability to produce collagen. Collagen gives skin density and youthful elastin which keeps our skin taut and elastic and moisture loss and loss of hyaluronic acid follows.

The Gene Mutation That Causes Progerin

A single gene mutation is responsible for progeria. The gene, known as Lamin A (LMNA), makes a protein necessary for holding the center (nucleus) of a cell together. When this gene has a defect (mutation), an abnormal form of the lamin A protein called progerin is produced and makes cells unstable and causes signs of aging in skin.

Progerin And Aging Skin

Hyaluronic acid which hydrates our skin is what makes a baby's skin look plump. Excess progerin causes skin to wither, lose suppleness and become dry. As fat under the skin is destroyed through a process called lipoatrophy, that is when our faces become gaunt, jowly and lined.

UVA And Progerin

Research has found that exposure to UVA rays from the sun increases the amount of progerin our skin produces, which helps explain exactly why overzealous tanning prematurely ages the skin. As it became clear that progerin is a key cause of aging, beauty companies were quick to spot an opportunity. If progerins could be removed from cells, it seemed possible to also reverse skin aging.

Dermal Filler Alternatives

Now cutting-edge research is helping to create a new generation of weapons in the war against wrinkles. The cosmetic giants realise that by focusing on Progerin products, with ingredients that block the toxic protein they can take some of the market that previously was only treatable with filler injections or surgery.

DMAE & Skin Tightening

Dimethylaminoethanol (DMAE) is a nutritional supplement that supports the saying that fish is brain food. DMAE is also one of the best options for tightening sagging jowls and eyelids and plumping gaunt cheeks and temples, as well as reducing wrinkles. Numerous studies have shown that topical application of DMAE increases the appearance of firmness, tone and lift to the skin. DMAE also improves the appearance of skin elasticity and luminosity, helping to decrease the look of fine lines and wrinkles while brightening skin's appearance and evening out imperfections. DMAE is naturally produced in the body. It's also found in some foods.

Foods High In DMAE:

- fatty fish
- salmon,
- sardines,
- anchovies.

Marine Algae- Topical Anti-Wrinkle Compound That Works

The only topical face creams and serums that really work are those that contain marine algae extract, researchers claim it makes progerins self-destruct and be eliminated from skin cells.

Marine algae is one of the most abundant sources of vitamins, minerals, amino acids, antioxidants and essential fatty acids that are readily absorbed to nourish and rejuvenate the skin. In general, algae are known to contain proteins and amino acids that aid in the production of collagen, and rich in Omega-3 fatty acids needed for various health benefits, including but not limited to, reducing skin damage.

Algae extract is from four major seaweed classes:

- red algae,
- brown algae,
- blue-green algae, and
- green algae.

Each class of algae contains molecules that promote skin benefits such as:

- omega 3 fatty acids,
- amino acids,
- vitamins A, B, C, and E.

Chapter 15

Causes Of External Signs Of Aging & Solutions

Chronological aging accounts for close to 20 percent of the signs of aging the other 80% consist of factors that cause external aging are:

- UV damage
- Stress and
- Pollution

While you can prevent sun damage by avoiding too much sun exposure, it was long thought that we couldn't prevent intrinsic aging. However, scientific research indicates that by helping cells to eliminate progerin we can also fight chronological aging, too.

Many labs are developing topical progerin blockers for skincare. Omega Statine and Z-Dronate are two patented topical active ingredients found in the oral drug used to treat progeria, the age accelerator disease that makes little children look old and age rapidly. Now, these Progerin blocker substances have been micronised so they can penetrate into the skin. Product manufacturers claim that by applying the micronized solutions may make the bad progerin protein less toxic and additionally, they may help slow the rate of aging in the skin to kickstart cell renewal and collagen production. The clinical trials showed a reduction in the worst form of wrinkles, deep wrinkles.

Algae Bad Progerin Protein & Wrinkle Eliminator

An Algae extract, Alaria Esculenta, has an inhibitory effect on the bad, wrinkle-causing protein, progerin.

An Algae Extract Suppresses Progerin & Helps Prevent Wrinkles

Alaria Esculenta, known as:

- Dabberlocks,
- Badderlocks,
- Winged Kelp or
- Atlantic Wakame,

Alaria, is a seaweed found on the coasts of the Irish Atlantic. Unlike Japanese wakame, which is often blanched, Irish Alaria is dark green. If you choose to include Alaria in your diet, choose a source, not in the region of the Fukushima nuclear meltdown, research the source for obvious reasons. Irish sourced is prefered in today's markets and in its natural state.

As a whole food, Alaria's delicate dark green leaf is delicious and beautiful addition to your:

- soups,
- salads and
- stir fries

Alaria algae is rich in nutrition:

- amino acids
- powerful antioxidants
- vitamins and
- minerals

Alaria also contains:

- Vitamin A, B, K
- Fiber
- Magnesium
- Iron
- Potassium
- Iodine
- Chlorophyll (great for detoxification)

Alaria Esculenta it helps:

- Increase skin firmness
- Decrease wrinkles
- Detoxifying the body and skin
- Energizes the skin.
- Increases blood circulation
- Improves thyroid function

This makes Alaria a key substance for radiant health and youthful-looking skin. It helps with:

- collagen-enhancing,
- moisturising and
- superior hydrating abilities,

Independent research studies found:

- Alaria slows production of the bad protein, progerin
- Alaria blocks progerin production in cells
- Alaria can make skin 25% firmer
- Alaria can make skin 20% more elastic
- Alaria topical essential extract helps reduce wrinkles

Look for the following ingredients in your skin care products for the purpose of eliminating progerin and lifting sagging skin.

Anti-Progerin Compounds:

Alaria Esculenta- natural sea kelp extract some man-made altered natural substances that help neutralize progerin are;

- Actiprogerin- claims to limit progerin synthesis in skin cells.
- Progeline- mimics elafin, a natural protein.
- Elafin-blocks the production of progerin and protects elastin
- Supports healthy elastin in skin that keeps it tight and firm.

Progerin Shortens Telomeres

Our telomeres are tiny "caps" on the ends of our chromosomes that shorten as we grow older. It has been discovered that this shortening of telomeres also triggers the production of progerin, the bad protein that causes wrinkles and aging in our skin.

Progerin Blockers

Alaria esculenta seaweed, helps prevent progerin and it has long been eaten fresh or cooked in nordic countries such as:

- Greenland,
- Iceland,
- Scotland and
- Ireland.

Food Categories:

- Alariaceae
- Sea vegetables

There are twelve species of Alaria. Here are some food extracts that boost the length of our telomeres that contain Alaria.

- Atlantic Wakame Seaweed
- Dabberlocks or
- Badderlocks
- Láir or Láracha (in Ireland)

The extracts and oils from this algae can also be used as an additive in various other food products or as an oil replacement for salads and other foods.

These types of kelp are the ones to take for beauty and anti-aging. Increasing your intake of Alaria Esculenta is a fantastic way to reap the skin-boosting properties of antioxidants. The nutrient-rich sea kelp is an anti-progerin ingredient in many skincare products, including anti-aging brand anti-wrinkle cream.

Elafin Is The Progerin Blocker In Alaria

Progeline is a 3 amino acid peptide biomimetic of elafin that has a unique mechanism of action on progerin synthesis and modulation. By acting directly on this new senescence marker, Progeline clinically reduces signs of skin aging in the following ways:

- Reduces sagging and
- Reduces wrinkles
- Improves firmness
- Improves Elasticity
- Jawline contour
- Neck Skin tightening

Chapter 16

Tips To Activate Your Inner Fountain Of Youth

The Secret To Activating Your Inner Fountain Of Youth

The most important thing to age youthfully and activate your inner fountain of youth is by following a sensible daily age reversing protocol that will help you better control the way you age. These basics can not only prevent and reverse chronic illnesses but also the signs and symptoms of aging.

Key Tips To Activate Your Inner Fountain Of Youth

Activating your inner fountain of youth doesn't have to be an overwhelming task. It can be as simple as changing the things you do to yourself because the damage that we do to ourselves with bad habits, are the easiest things to correct. There are a number of ways that you can activate your body's self-healing mechanisms and optimize your health while prolonging the time left on your biological clock to extend your life-span.

- **Step One** The first step of the reverse aging program deals with making dietary changes, boosting the immune system, reducing systemic inflammation and removing toxic waste from the body- all pretty basic stuff. In other words, this part of the damage control is up to you. You are in charge and play an active role in how effectively you can reverse aging, but more about that in the other chapters.

  - **Put Your Phone Down**
    With today's 5G towers and technology concerns, it is even more important that we take frequent breaks from our phones. Phones are an essential part of any working day; we take them everywhere and put them down everywhere. Your trusty phones and gadgets that you touch and often hold to your face several times a day are loaded with more bacteria than a toilet. Additionally, your mobile phone emits blue

light and is a source of bacteria, both of which can cause pigmentation and wrinkles, so choose a sunscreen that includes zinc oxide, which is known to offer wide-ranging protection

- **Electronic Smog From Technology**
  If you spend hours working at your computer, the screen time could be adding years to your skin through the invisible electronic smog, that is as damaging as UV rays. There is newly emerging evidence that the light from computer screens and cell phones, which is referred to as high-energy visible light (HEV) can penetrate into the deeper levels of the skin. This results in free radical damage that can break down skin collagen and elastin, the structures that keep the skin firm and youthful, leading to the development of fine lines and wrinkles not to mention sagging skin.

- **Stop Smoking & Avoid Exposure**
  Everyone knows smoking is bad for your health, but it's also very bad for your skin. Kick the habit of smoking! It seriously damages your looks as it accelerates aging and lowers collagen production by up to 22 percent.

- **Step Two** The second part of damage control involves preventing and reversing damage at the cellular level. This component of reverse aging may not totally be up to you as factors promoting aging are genetically programmed in your cells. Having said that, there arc still some proactive measures you can take to prevent damage at the cellular level.

  - you can incorporate more exercise into your daily routine to keep circulation moving, the heart pumping well, and the lymphatic system flowing freely. This will, among other things, nourish and replenish your cells well.
  - you can invest in some quality anti-aging products that will work internally to regenerate cells and minimize aging effects. A lot more on this in upcoming chapters.

- **Step Three** The final step in this process addresses hormonal changes that affect aging at a macro level. Hormones are the body's chemical messengers telling the body what to do and when and with regards to aging, hormones tell the body how to age and fluctuations in hormonal levels does affect aging.

  - While hormonal production cannot be completely dominated by any single treatment, you can make small but sensible changes to restore

these imbalances. Some basics to boost the body's ability to create and balance hormones include changing lifestyle and dietary habits while staying away from common stressors and detoxifying.
  ○ Consider hormonal balancing therapy.

- **Get Your Beauty Sleep**

  Eight hours of sleep really can help you look and feel your best. As you sleep many beauty restoring regeneration processes happen in your body as soon as you drift off. The truth about beauty sleep is that while you're sleeping, your body and your skin are hard at work healing themselves. During the deeper phases of sleep, your body produces growth hormone, which repairs daily damage from things like sun exposure and pollution and creates new cells so you wake up looking brighter, fresher, and more vibrant. That's why bedtime can be a great time to apply a night cream to help accelerate the restorative process.

  - ○ Fewer Wrinkles.
  - ○ Skin makes new collagen when you sleep,
  - ○ Prevents sagging.
  - ○ Rested Glowing Complexion.
  - ○ Your body boosts blood flow to the skin while you snooze.
  - ○ A healthy glow.
  - ○ Brighter Eyes
  - ○ Less Bags & Puffy Eyes.
  - ○ Refreshed Feeling
  - ○ Happier Mood
  - ○ Healthier Appearance.

Moods & Facial Aging

For starters, when people are sad and frowning all the time, eventually facial muscles sag due to daily facial expression. When a person is depressed, they aren't smiling as much and when you smile you flex hundreds of muscles and tone them. Various moods from sadness to anger may cause a tensing of specific facial muscles, grimacing or frowning, and these "negative facial expressions can become sort of etched into the skin in the form of fine lines and wrinkles, especially around the lips, and lower jowls.

Stress & Facial Aging

Stress can cause wrinkles to form because high amounts of cortisol, the stress hormone, can break down the skin's collagen and elastin. Research has found that chronic stress can increase inflammation, causing skin aging and accelerating the formation of wrinkles.

How To Keep Your Face From Sagging

Avoiding smoking, stressful life events and eating a diet rich in fruit and vegetables are two lifestyle factors which can make a big difference. The products you choose can also stop skin sagging from becoming any more severe. Always wear sunscreen and an SPF of at least factor SPF 30, to protect against UV rays.

This is a new science so you will need to follow updates as they develop and are discover to find the latest ingredient that work to deactivate the effects of progerin, it is an ongoing research to find the magic anti-aging compound but anti-progerin ingredients tend to be expensive and results are not yet comparable to dermal fillers or surgery. However, the research is still very new and improvements are being made all the time but for those who don't fret with cost, for results that are natural, subtle and needle and knife-free anti-progerin products are the best option for home skin care maintenance as is found in anti-aging skin rx brand.

Age Blocker Pills

Anti-Aging is not about taking antioxidants or human growth hormone and it's not only about exercise and eating a healthy diet, though all these things help. The closest thing to a "magic-pill" for anti-aging are the dietary supplements:

- NAD
- NMN
- NR

AMPK Activation & Stimulation

At the molecular level aging is not just about free-radical damage, the reason why we age is because protein can't get into the cell and the body withers when our info dwindles as the telomeres shorten as we age to the point of death. NAD+ helps DNA write the correct combination of Genetic and Epigenetic information without errors helps repair DNA and our bodies. The genome is four bases of a binary way of preserving our genetic information.

Collagen Protein COL17A1

Collagen Type XVII Alpha 1 is a protein coding gene. The collagen protein called COL17A1 plays a key role in maintaining youthful skin. Declining levels of this protein over time cause our skin to develop wrinkles, sag, and lose its elasticity. Skin continually rebuilds itself and produces new cells. COL17A1 is instrumental in stronger skin cells and helps skin rebuild itself and produce new cells.

- Improves skin regeneration and can fight aging and speed up wound healing

Apocynin Anti Skin Cancer Agent

Apocynin Rho kinase inhibitor Y27632 promotes proliferation of human keratinocytes but not fibroblasts or squamous cell carcinoma (SCC) of the skin, the second most common form of skin cancer, characterized by abnormal, accelerated growth of squamous cells. Helps healthy new skin to regenerate.

Sulforaphane Super Anti-Aging Compound

The natural antioxidant sulforaphane, found in broccoli, exerts anticarcinogenic, antidiabetic and antimicrobial properties. Sulforaphane extracts applied topically protects skin against UVR-induced inflammation and edema and is a powerful anti-aging compound.

"Bad" Foods That Are Good For You

1. **Fruit**- whole fruit is not bad for you. It is loaded with more anti-aging compounds than most other foods, all the vitamins, minerals, bioflavonoids and fiber your body needs can be found in raw whole fruits.
2. **Coffee & Tea** - organic, hot or cold, these beverages contain antioxidants that the typical american diet is lacking. Drink up! A cup a day may help keep the doctor away.
3. **Fats**- fatty acids are good for anti-aging skin, joints and brain. Too much of a good thing becomes a bad thing. Limit your intake to 1-2 tablespoons a day. Avoid cooking foods in fat.
4. **Eggs**- the omegas, lecithin, protein is unsurpassable. Eggs are a superfood, but again, not too many. Hormone free and free-range eggs are good for you. If you only have an egg only a few times a week they are good for you. Avoid frying.
5. **Veggie Pizza**- all organic non gmo gluten free or with a cauliflower crust, is probably one of the healthiest dishes on the planet, in moderation.

"Good" Foods That Aren't Really Good

Many foods labeled healthy food, are loaded with other bad things to compensate for the lack of flavor from the missing ingredients, such as some foods labeled:

- Fat free- these foods are usually loaded with salt or sugar
- Sugar free- these foods are usually loaded with even more dangerous artificial sweeteners
- Diet - loaded with salt and artificial flavors and fillers.

The Key To Eating Is Moderation

Being Obese Ages You

Obesity accelerates the aging process more than smoking, according to the biggest study ever done on the "chromosomal clock" in human cells. A study in epigenetics revealed that obesity accelerates epigenetic changes associated with aging in the human liver resulting in an apparent age acceleration of 2.7 years for a 10-point increase in BMI. Therefore, obesity triggers other comorbidities that decrease mortality rate and life expectancy and is now classified as a disease that requires a multidisciplinary healthcare approach including medical, dietary and psychological treatment.

Obesity symptoms include:

- Bulging fatty pockets
- Breathlessness.
- Overeating wrong foods
- Increased sweating.
- Decreased agility
- Snoring.
- Exhaustion with physical activity.
- Increased risk of back and joint pains & injury.
- Low confidence
- Lack of self esteem.
- Feeling discriminated, judged, isolated.
- Higher risk for diabetes and other obesity related diseases.

Healthy Weight Management- Those who are a few pounds overweight but with a healthy BMI can often lose those excess pounds and keep them off by following a healthy diet and lifestyle. Exercising regularly and eating a balanced diet, supplemented with high quality nutritional supplements and drinking water should be your first steps to maintaining good health. You can expect improvements such as:

- Increased oxygen levels
- Better blood sugar levels
- Better blood pressure
- Balanced appetite
- A better functioning body
- Lean muscle gains
- Fat and weight loss
- More energy and less fatigue

There are some natural substances that are clinically proven to promote effective weight loss:

- 5-HTP
- Flaxseed Oil
- Fucus Vesiculosus
- Green Tea Extract
- Guarana
- Zinc Pyruvate

Food Portion Control

The power of weight loss is in your hands when you control the foods you eat.

- **Carbohydrates-** avoid high carb counts by liminiting foods like processed white rice, instant oats, whit bread, wheat posta, instant potatoes and processed grains like grits.
- **Protein-** The recommended serving size of meat is 3 0z. Roughly the size of your palm.
- **Dairy-** A healthy portion of hormone free A2 dairy is 1 cup of skim milk or a palm size portion of sliced cheese or 1 tablespoon of parmesan cheese which is about 10-20 calories.
- **Fruits & Vegetables-** a proper serving of vegetables is about the size of your open hand. Fill your plate with a variety of different collared fruits and vegetables to ensure a wide array of nutrients in your diet.

179

- **Fatty Foods & Sugars**- Your fingertip is equal to about a teaspoon, which is how much butter you should spread on your toast, you can double this portion size for healthier fats such as avocado or peanut butter.
- **Sugar**- Limit sugary drinks, sweets, toppings and avoid foods with high fructose corn syrup or high sugar content.
- **Avoid Emotional Eating**- Find healthier activities and things to keep your mind and body busy rather than munching. Avoid emotional eating and binging on comfort foods or alcohol which are high in calories and for the most part unhealthy.
- **Bad Eating Habits**- Junk food junkie. This behavior is similar to addictive behaviors of a drug user, which is often referred to as a junkie when the person has no control over their use. Junk food junkies may require counseling to overcome and prevent food addictions. Also, read my book Quit or Die.

Eye Aging Prevention

As we grow older, often we will experience eye health changes. Many people have the need for reading glasses after the age of 40. One thing you can do to slow the degeneration of your eyes is N-Acetyl Cysteine (NAC). Research shows eyesight treated with NAC substantially improved within 6 months. The documented eye improvements of NAC include:

- 42% increase of transmissivity of the lenses
- 90% visual acuity improvement
- 89% glare sensitivity improvement

Carnosine Eye Drops

Applying carnosine eye drops according to the manufacturers label and gently pat any excess around the eye area into the lines or crows feet as carnosine also helps prevent wrinkles and cataracts among other eye health benefits.

Restore Skin Elasticity

- Collagen supplements.
- Collagen is a protein found in the skin's connective tissues.
- Retinol and retinoids. Retinol is a form of vitamin A.
- Hyaluronic acid.
- Genistein isoflavones.
- Hormone replacement therapy (HRT)

- Witch hazel extract.
- Cocoa flavanols.
- Laser treatments.

Age Prevention Super Supplements

While many of the anti-aging supplements may be available in stores, it may be more convenient or affordable to shop for them online:

- Astragalus
- Collagen
- CoQ10
- Curcumin
- EGCG
- Fisetin
- Green Tea
- Garlic (Kyolic)
- L-Theanine
- Rhodiola
- Resveratrol
- NMN
- NR
- Turmeric

Acetyl-L-Carnitine (NAC) is the biologically active form of the amino acid L-carnitine and has been shown to protect cells throughout the body against age-related degeneration. Most clinical research has focused on the brain, where improved mood, memory and cognition has been observed in response to acetyl-L-carnitine administration. By facilitating the youthful transport of fatty acids into the cell's mitochondria, acetyl-L-carnitine better enables dietary fats to be converted to energy and muscle.

NAC Key Benefits:
- Supports Cognitive Health
- Supports Energy Production
- Supports Cardiovascular Health
- Supports Cellular Energy Production

Carnitine

Carnitine is an amino-acid that protects against muscle wasting diseases, including heart muscle weakness and low energy levels. In addition, acetyl-L-carnitine is shown to maintain immune competence and reduce the cell-clogging pigment called lipofuscin that blocks the pathways of your inner fountain of youth. The most important anti-aging effect of acetyl-L-carnitine, is to work with coenzyme Q10 and alpha lipoic acid to maintain the function of the mitochondria. When mitochondria function dwindles, degenerative disease becomes an inevitable consequence. Acetyl-L-carnitine is a multi-purpose anti-aging supplement that also helps with brain function and brain anti-aging.

Acetyl-L-Carnitine

In the early 1980s, acetyl-L-carnitine (ALC) was approved as a "drug" in Europe to treat heart and neurological disease. Americans had to wait until 1994 to legally buy acetyl-L-carnitine. Since this amino acid is sold as a dietary supplement, it is a safe anti-aging supplement with many youthful benefits.

Chapter 17

Bad Habits That Speed Aging & Changes To Make To Slow Aging

Phasing Out Destructive Habits & Longevity Killers

We have covered the basics and you have anti-aging methods and ideals in place. Now that you know why aging happens it's time to learn how you may benefit from making daily age-reversing lifestyle choices. It is time to look at implementing changes that will actually help you reverse the aging process. Since everyone doesn't age the same way. In fact, there are a number of reasons why the pace at which each individual ages is different from anyone else. One way that you could be speeding up your aging process is by certain lifestyle choices that you make, more specifically, the bad habits that are injurious to your health in many ways. If you have any of the following bad habits, you are only fast-forwarding your aging and now is the time to quit or die from some horrible side effect related to the health detriment these habits cause:

- **Not Drinking Enough Water**

Water is the primary component in your inner fountain of youth. Dehydration is longevity's worst enemy. Water also contributes to regular bowel function, optimal muscle performance, and clear, youthful-looking skin. However, failing to drink enough water can cause dehydration and adverse symptoms, including fatigue, headache, weakened immunity, and dry skin.

"It Is Better To Be Full Of Drink Than Full Of Food" Hypocrites

- ## Smoking & Bad Air Quality Exposure

Smoking of any sort or form adversely affects almost every biological system in your body. It is no secret how it affects the lungs; damaging lung tissue, obstructing air passages and rendering lung tissues incapable of performing their main function: the exchange of oxygen with the inhaled air. It is this very oxygen that the blood carries to all the tissues to keep them healthy and active. This also includes the skin. If the oxygen is compromised, the body will automatically provide the bulk of it to the vital organs (brain, heart and liver), instead of the skin. With this poor supply of oxygen to the skin, the epidermis of the skin is unable to keep healthy or to regenerate. It can no longer form adequate proteins such as collagen, which is the main factor responsible for the elasticity of youthful and healthy skin.

As a result, in combination with bad proteins such as progerin, you get wrinkles, dry and damaged skin that make you look years older than your age. All the irritants in smoke harm various tissues and organ systems. Some of their unpleasant visible effects on aging is that they cause the white part of the eye, nails, and teeth to yellow, dull and lose their natural color. Giving up smoking can greatly help in reversing aging.

- ## Alcohol Consumption

Alcohol is ethanol, consumption of alcohol is similar to drinking gas, although the chemicals in gasoline are so toxic that if you drink it your kidneys would shut down and you would die. Alcohol is perhaps one of the worst age accelerators in the human diet. If you want to keep your inner fountain of youth flowing eliminate alcohol consumption from your lifestyle. ALcohol dehydrates your skin and damages every organ inside out, it is a destroyer to looking and feeling young. Too much alcohol can easily make a person in their 20's, look like forty- thin, weak, pale, bags under the eyes coupled with the overall neurotic behaviour and mental breakdowns. The effects Alcohol consumption has on aging goes much deeper than just skin. Read my book "Quit or Die, The Truth About Alcohol" The organs most affected by alcohol are the brain, liver, kidneys and skin. Alcohol kills! Read Quit or Die to find out why.

- ## Illicit Drugs

Drugs are chemical compounds. The liver is a vital organ, and its failure could potentially lead to death. One of the functions of the liver is to detoxify the body. As drugs and alcohol are processed as toxins, the liver has to work extra hard to remove them from the system. Excessive drug use and alcohol consumption will exhaust liver cells so they are unable to function. Not only does alcohol increase physiological toxicity, but the failure of the liver to fight chemical toxins will speed up the process of aging years.

- **Sugar Intake**

White sugar is the most toxic and addictive food on the planet. It is very common to associate sugar intake with obesity, diabetes and other health issues. But it is less common knowledge that sugar fastens your aging process as well. Glucose, the simplest form of sugar, is the main substrate for energy in the body but the wrong can can convert to alcohol in the body and cause the same type of damage and in excess can lead to a number of diabetic like type complications. It can cause wrinkles by dehydrating the skin and can also cause dark circles to appear under the eyes like a drug addict. Additionally, glucose metabolism produces AGEs (Advanced Glycation End products). Appropriately named, AGEs can disrupt DNA replication to fail causing your skin to age quickly and look old and saggy. A high sugar intake will age more than just the skin. All the organs have to work more to metabolise that extra sugar and will exhaust much faster than the normal, natural pace of aging. While healthy levels of glucose are extremely important for the body, its excess will most certainly age you faster.

- **Emotional Eating**

When people feel anxious and bored and get caught up in stressful emotions, the stress hormones change your chemistry and metabolism, immediately and it can turn food into stored fat, quickly and trigger a metabolic imbalance. Those that may be more likely to become vulnerable to emotional eating for comfort should see a therapist as this type of eating has similarities to drug addiction.

- **Sedentary Sitting Too Much**

In this day and age, most of our day involves sitting down for hours. Be it working in an office, studying in an academic setting, or even just sitting and doing nothing at all, there is too much sitting going on in the day. Whether you are being productive or not, sitting for hours can cause aging to creep up on you.

More specifically, epidemiological evidence proves that those who sit for more than 10 hours a day age 8 years faster. Imagine, being only 30 and looking 38. Or being 40 and looking 48! Petty scary stuff, most would agree. This is why you must try to move around as much as possible. Forget the elevator, take the stairs. Never mind the shortcut, walk the longer route home. Make sure to move around every hour even if you have piles of work at your desk. This will help counter aging effectively.

- **Binge Watching and Binge Eating**

Bad news for all those who binge watch- it can make you age faster! There is actually a thing called 'The Netflix Face' by experts. This is characterised by wrinkles, spots and fine lines. The screens of mobile phones, laptops and other devices emit harmful radiation that penetrate into the skin and damage it.

Like previous lifestyles mentioned above, this one also does not stop at the skin alone. Binge watchers should be wary, because this bad habit is causing their brains to age faster too. It can greatly affect different functions of the brain, causing attention deficits, concentration deficits, bad memory, and slower processing and comprehension of information.

Binge watching and binge eating are a bad combination which, if not controlled, can be very dangerous for health. Avoiding it will help you age slower.

- **Poor Posture**

While this does not exactly show signs of aging on the face, it does so inside the body. The posture affects how well blood is being pumped in the body and also how well a person breathes.

For someone who is used to "slumping" all the time, straightening up will immediately reveal what a difference good posture makes. An upright and erect posture is very important in controlling aging. Bad postures lead to problems that are mostly seen in adults and are now experienced by youngsters. For example, back aches, pain in joints and breathlessness. It is important to maintain good posture at all times to avoid the development of such signs of aging.

- **Using The 'Wrong' Makeup**

We all love the difference that makeup can make to your appearance and confidence, it is also one of the biggest culprits in premature aging. The internet is loaded with tutorials that show a person putting on layers upon layers of makeup but they are often using cheap brands that are loaded with chemicals, plastics, alcohol and other carcinogens. Wearing makeup comes hand-in-hand with the removal and properly cleansing it off of your skin each night.

This is why the brand you choose is important, you will be safe choosing a brand that is all natural with clean ingredients without the chemicals that are common in many store bought brands. We prefer the Anti-Aging Brand makeup and Anti-Aging Skin Rx skincare. The skincare and makeup is all natural, high quality with super anti-aging benefits. Anti-Aging brand started out in Hollywood and was designed by celebrity skincare specialist, as when they are filming onset the cast, crew and directors are constantly exposed to the heat and harsh lighting of set photography lighting, additionally they are exposed to high levels of free-radicals from the radiation of all the film equipment and bright lights. Yet they often appear to be ageless and possess super beauty. If you've ever wondered how they do it, it's because of the beauty professionals they go to when they're off set. A celebrities behind the scenes narrative is keeping up their appearance and good health. Because after all, their real job is to keep themselves in tip-top shape so they can work as long as possible. In the past an actor was considered washup after 30 years old in Hollywood, that is no longer the case, 50 is the new 20 in Hollywood and it is because they have had access to these compounds immediately upon discovery in the ivy league medical research labs across the globe. Now we can get these compounds more easily and at reasonable prices so that the rest of the populations can enjoy in-home anti-aging, too.

Toxic Personal Care Products

Most commercial products contain waxes, chemicals, emulsifiers and alcohol that will rob your skin of its natural moisture and components, dehydrate it and contribute to the causes of wrinkles. Applying the wrong makeup and not properly cleansing from your skin makes you age many times faster. To avoid this, it is important to use good quality, natural makeup and as minimally as possible and avoid the following bad habits:

- Smoking
- Over Drinking
- Excess Sun Exposure
- Eating AGE's Junk Food
- Lack Of Exercise

Restore Skin Elasticity

- Collagen supplement.
  - Collagen is a protein found in the skin's connective tissues that we lose as we age.

- Retinol and retinoids.
  - Retinol is a form of topical vitamin A.

- Hyaluronic acid.
  - The hydration in the skin and joints that dehydrates with age.

- Genistein isoflavones.
  - Boost the immune system

- Hormone replacement therapy (HRT)
  - Replacement of the hormones that decline with age.

- Witch hazel extract.
  - Tones and tightens surface skin

- Cocoa flavanols.
  - Cacao is an excellent source of age fighting antioxidants

- Laser treatments.
  - Exfoliates off dead dry surface layers and tightens sagging tissue with controlled heat.

Anti-aging therapies are beneficial for longer lasting youthful looking beauty and for the life-long maintenance of a healthy body.

Nobody Wants To Look Old

People invest a lot of money, time and energy to avoid looking and feeling old. The appearance of the first wrinkle or grey hair can be quite distressing. Anti-Aging treatments can give your confidence and self-esteem a boost. You look the way you feel. If you feel younger from the inside, you will look younger on the outside, too. It is not just the skin that needs to look vibrant and young to make you feel better about yourself. Taking better care of yourself helps eliminate insecurities and can relieve many health worries.

Obesity Accelerates Aging

Obesity is a massive problem in our population. The comorbidities of obesity are linked to a huge burden of diseases including:

- high blood pressure,
- heart disease,
- cancers,
- reproductive problems, and
- diabetes.

In fact, an estimated 80% of diabetes would not exist in the absence of obesity.

Excess cortisol causes a build-up of belly fat. So the researchers thought this might be the reason why certain people tend to develop a "beer belly" while others don't. They looked at an enzyme called 11-beta hydroxysteroid dehydrogenase type 1. This enzyme is able to increase the level of cortisol in fat cells without raising the level of cortisol in the blood.

Cortisol

Cortisol is a stress hormone responsible for the "fight or flight" mode we experience during extreme stress. The cortisol hormone kicks in during all stressful situations and it stops your digestion and metabolism shifting the body's metabolic energies to the brain and extremities so your body can fight or flee a threatening situation without having to stop to go to the bathroom while your running away from a tiger or struggling to survive a car-crash or a battle of some sort. The problem is, your body can't tell the difference between psychological or physiological stress, your body treats both types of stress in the same response. Literally, your body mechanisms act the same regardless if you're having a fight with someone over who's taking the garbage out or if you're having a fight for your life with an animal that's trying to attack and eat you. When the body produces excess cortisol, regardless of the reason, it tends to cause a build-up of belly fat. Recently, researchers sought to find out why certain people tend to develop beer-belly type weight gain.

They discovered an enzyme called:

- 11-beta hydroxysteroid dehydrogenase type 1 (HSD1).
- The HSD1 enzyme increases the level of cortisol in fat cells that overtime, results in an accumulation of abdominal fat.
- HSD1) activates glucocorticoid locally in liver and fat tissues to aggravate metabolic syndrome.

- Effective selective inhibitors of HSD1 are:

    o Hormone balancers and stabilizers
    o Terpenoids
    o Flavonoids

Chapter 18

How To Repair The Effects Of Bad Habits

Choices After A Life Of Toxins

Many people have lived a life full of bad habits and have unintentionally filled their bodies full of toxins during the process. When we are young and healthy it doesn't seem to affect us to have hotdogs and beer for breakfast, but at some point if you continue these bad habits, you will eventually wake up feeling like crap and a smart person will decide to clean their life up and get healthy again. The not-so-smart will continue their health decline until they have a heart-attack or develop diabetes before they decide to quit or die. The others will eventually die younger than they would have and usually from some god-awful condition.

You are obviously one of the smart people who have decided to clean up their bad habits thus the reason you're reading this book. The good news is, it is not too late. Here's what you can do to get healthy and activate your inner fountain of youth.

If You Live Better You Will Live Longer

If you have lived a high stress, unhappy or junk-food lifestyle there are some steps you can take to offset the damage caused to your inner fountain of youth to begin turning your health around. One of the main causes of death is the buildup of old cells and bad cell proteins that block the good proteins from getting into the cells and doing their job.

Take Systemic Enzymes

Systemic enzymes to help your liver break down and eliminate metabolic waste

- Serrapeptase

- Nattokinase
- Trypsin
- Proteolytic Enzymes
- And more

These valuable forms of systemic enzymes will help activate your inner fountain of youth by getting rid of stagnation and waking up cells stimulating active enzyme activity. These enzymes have the ability to break down the old metabolic waste to get rid of plaque, arthritic deposits in joints, inflammation, dead cellular debris, scar tissue, stagnation and sludge buildup like a spring cleaning, year round.

Cortisol, Fat & Starch Blockers For Weight Loss

- **Starch Blockers**

    Starch Blockers work mainly on an enzyme in your saliva to help slow down the process by which the complex carbohydrate and starchy foods are absorbed and are known as alpha-glucosidase inhibitors (AGIs). Carb blockers do not block all of the cabs, they only prevent a portion of the carbohydrates that you eat from being absorbed. AGI's are widely used in the treatment of patients with type 2 diabetes. AGIs help block the absorption of carbohydrates from the small intestine and thus have a lowering effect on postprandial blood glucose and insulin levels.

The benefits of carb blockers include the following:

- Improves blood sugar levels
- May help weight loss
- May help curb your appetite
- Prevents some of the absorption of carb
- Sugar consumption is not blocked by AGIs

Natural sources effective for blocking carbohydrates:

- White kidney bean extract - white bean extract from the common bean, green bean and French bean are known to inhibit the digestive enzyme alpha-amylase, which may prevent the digestion of complex carbohydrates and may result in wcight loss.
- Salacia plants- Salacia is an herb classified as a woody climber naturally found in tropical regions. Several species in this genus have been used in traditional medicine, such as the Ayurvedic system from India. The root and stem are

used to make tea or medicine. Salacia has a long history of use for treatments in traditional Indian medicine. Salacia is used for treating obesity.

Fat Blockers

There's only one proven fat blocker that's over-the-counter and FDA-approved. Orlistat which is also marketed as Alli and Xenical. These block 25% of fat that people consume according to the studies.

Best Diet, Exercise & Behavior Modification Plan

In a randomized study of 250 healthy patients in conjunction with a multi-component weight-loss program, including diet, exercise, and behavioral modification. We used the healthy diet and weight loss program exactly as outlined in "The Balance Diet And Lifestyle" book by Joyce Peters and Summer Perry. We followed 200 patients for 3 months and then conducted a one year maintenance checkup. The results showed that 75% of all participants reduced their weight by an average of 9-11 pounds within 3 months and the remaining 25% had reduced their weight and waist size significantly. The average weight loss was 15 pounds and 3" off the waistline, within 6 months. 25 of the participants were followed for the subsequent 3 years with an annual checkup concluded that all of those who adhered to the healthy lifestyle program kept the weight off for more than 3 years. The Balance Diet and Lifestyle program includes dietary modification, exercise, and behavioral intervention, the study concluded that a healthy lifestyle plan can significantly reduce excess weight and waist size in a short period of time and help you maintain a healthy weight long-term, longer than 3 years simply by following the Balance Diet and Lifestyle.

Exercise Is The Closest Thing To A Magic Best Anti-Aging Pill

Exercise helps your body eliminate excess fat and keep your metabolism in peak condition. Aerobic exercise is important for improving body functions and quality of life. Previous studies have demonstrated that aerobic exercise delays aging, the retardation of cognitive functions and the decline of neurological functions.

Antioxidants Vs. Good Fats For Anti-Aging

Taking antioxidants have long been touted for their anti-aging benefits. For the past decade, mice studies show conflicts about the most touted antioxidants. According to experts who have conducted massive amounts of government backed research in age research, scientists discovered that a high fat diet is detrimental to the anti-aging effects of resveratrol. The researchers found that a high-fat diet cancels out the anti-aging benefits of taking resveratrol. Therefore, it's not only important to take resveratrol for its anti-aging benefits, it is equally important to eat a healthy diet with good-fats and avoid a high-fat diet to reap all of the wonderful anti-aging benefits of resveratrol.

Sweat Off Excess Weight

Exercise helps you break a sweat. Daily movement can reduce excess fat and elevate your mood. Keep it simple, set aside the time daily, set your alarm and do it until you sweat. Drinking water during exercise will help you sweat more and sweat more quickly.

- Walking
- Jogging
- Cycling
- Jumping Jacks

Tighten Loose Skin During Weight Loss

As we age skin becomes loose from a loss of collagen and elastin in the skin. Taking collagen supplements and doing skin tightening treatments can help tighten skin. Walking and jogging stimulates the formation of collagen

Appetite Control

Leptin and Ghrelin control our hunger signals. Taking a hormone balancer can help with quelching and calming these hunger pains and hunger hormones. Mild vagus nerve exercises combined with supplemental amino acids and 5-HTP (5 hydroxytryptophan) helps increase your serotonin levels resulting in a decrease in appetite without drugs. In response to food intake, entero endocrine cells secrete gut hormones, which ultimately suppress appetite. Increasing evidence implicates the vagus nerve is an important conduit in transmitting these signals from the gastrointestinal tract to the brain. Freezing the vagus nerve could be therapeutic as a weight-loss tool.

Age Blocker Pills

Anti-Aging is not about taking antioxidants or human growth hormone and it's not only about exercise and eating a healthy diet, though all these things help. The closest thing to a "magic-pill" for anti-aging are the dietary supplements:

- NAD
- NMN
- NR

AMPK Activation & Stimulation

At the molecular level aging is not just about free-radical damage, the reason why we age is because protein can't get into the cell and the body withers when our info dwindles as the telomeres shorten as we age to the point of death. NAD+ helps DNA write the correct combination of Genetic and Epigenetic information without errors helps repair DNA and our bodies. The genome is four bases of a binary way of preserving our genetic information.

Antioxidants Vs. Good Fats For Anti-Aging

Taking antioxidants have long been touted for their anti-aging benefits. For the past decade, mice studies show conflicts about the most touted antioxidants. According to experts who have conducted massive amounts of government backed research in age research, scientists discovered that a high fat diet is detrimental to the anti-aging effects of resveratrol. The researchers found that a high-fat diet cancels out the anti-aging benefits of taking resveratrol. Therefore, it's not only important to take resveratrol for its anti-aging benefits, it is equally important to eat a healthy diet with good-fats and avoid a high-fat diet to reap all of the wonderful anti-aging benefits of resveratrol.

Anti-Aging Lifestyle Habits:

1. Exercise (daily & avoid being sedentary)
2. Diet (intermittent fasting)
3. Stay Hungry (never eat till full)
4. Stay Cold (keep home temp around 60)
5. FIR Sauna (Detox)
6. Baths (Stimulate)

Anti-Aging Regimen

- **Exercise-** at least 7 hours per week
- **Yoga-** movement is important
- **Walking-** daily
- **Sauna-** detox 3 x weekly
- **Hot Tub-** daily
- **Cold Bath-** 3-5 x weekly
- **Autophagy-** is the body's way of cleaning out dead or damaged cells, in order to regenerate newer, healthier cells "Auto" means self and "phagy" means eat. Autophagy is "self-eating."
- **Mind Set-** keep an outgoing social friendly mindset.
- **Mental health-** keep a check on your state of mental health and strive to stay in a state of good mental health.
- **Stress Management-** stress ages you. Get mental "stressors" out of your life.
- **Living In Love-** the vibration of love is very strengthening and healing, giving and receiving love is essential for happy life and longevity.
- **Good Diet-** the food you eat does support good health. You are what you eat.
- **Positive Thinking-** think positive and eliminate negativity
- **Subconscious Mind Awareness-** correct mis programming
- **Self-improvement** - look for ways to better yourself
- **Guided Meditations-** Visualization Techniques
- **Self-Hypnosis-** work on reprogramming for better habits.
- **Neurolinguistic Programming-** if you have negative or bad self talk change your thoughts to positive and healthy self-talk and learn to use your words to positively influence others.
- **Intermittent Fasting-** staying a little hungry is good

  - Not eating for 3 hours before bed & fast while you sleep

Bad Diet Advice

Many FAD diet advisors and authors have been proven to be wrong in their approaches to weight loss. Who wants to pay for good advice when you can get shitty advice for $1 and bad advice for free on the internet? The bottom line is if you can't get the weight off go see a specialist, being obese shorten's you lifespan and it's worth the money to get help to preserve your good health. Most overweight people have a metabolic imbalance that requires an interdisciplinary care approach, monitoring by a doctor, nutritionist, fitness trainer and psychologist. For more tips read "The Balance Diet and Lifestyle" by Joyce Peters

DNA blockers to avoid:

Mold/Mycotoxins
Yeast/Fungal Infections
Parasites
Bacterial infection
Good bacteria
Dirty Biofilm/Virome

Mood

If you are angry, worried, or in a hostile environment, no matter what else you do, your mood is aging you. Clean up your emotions, feelings or remove yourself from the environment that is stressing you and move into a better, healthier, more peaceful fun place.

Internet Fasting- yes, internet fasting! Our computers emit radiation plus surfing the internet keeps us from surfing the seas, and keeps us from getting out and in touch with mother. Getting back in touch with your own physical environment and people is important to good health.

Electro-Smog-

Our phones and computers emit electronic smog and radiation which is damaging to our DNA

DNA (deoxyribonucleic acid)

DNA is the hereditary material found in humans, animals, and organisms. DNA is in every cell in our bodies. Each cell's nucleus has DNA, which is rolled into structures that are our chromosomes (23 pairs)

Genes

Most genes contain the information needed to make functional molecules called proteins. A few genes produce other molecules that help the cell assemble proteins. The journey from gene to protein is complex and tightly controlled within each cell. It consists of two major steps:

- transcription

- translation

Together, transcription and translation are known as gene expression. During the process of transcription, the information stored in a gene's DNA is transferred to a similar molecule called RNA (ribonucleic acid) in the cell nucleus. Both RNA and DNA are made up of a chain of nucleotide bases, but they have slightly different chemical properties. The type of RNA that contains the information for making a protein is called messenger RNA (mRNA) because it carries the information, or message, from the DNA out of the nucleus into the cytoplasm.

The genes direct protein production. For example, a protein (a long chain of amino acids) can be an enzyme that triggers a certain chemical reaction in the body. One function of protein is to boost the immune system.

There are many factors that cause damaged DNA :

- oxidation,
- UV radiation from the sun,
- radiation from X Rays,
- viruses,
- mycotoxins
- plant toxins,
- man-made chemicals

    o chlorine,
    o hydrogen peroxide,
    o hydrocarbons,
    o smoke,
    o Pollution,
    o And more.

Some results of damaged DNA are:

- premature aging,
- cancer,
- diabetes mellitus
- diabetes itself may cause DNA damage
- parkinsons
- alzheimers
- chronic fatigue syndrome,

- and many other conditions.

Cells cannot function properly if the DNA is damaged. However, the cells can through chemical processes partially reverse the damage themselves.

Edestin DNA Repair

Hemp Protein and hemp seed oil have been found to be a factor in DNA repair. Hemp has the perfect 3:1 ratio of Omega fatty acids (Omega 3 and Omega 6) needed by the human body. One 'job' of Omega 3 is cellular repair. Hemp also has 65% globulin Edestin protein, which is very easily digestible by the body.

Edestin protein is a major factor in DNA repair, as the cells use that protein to correct the DNA damage.

Edestin Protein

Edestin is a highly-digestible, hexameric legumin protein. Edestin is similar to blood plasma, and the biologically active protein of edestin is metabolized in the human body and capable of bio synthesization of:

- Hormones- helps regulate all the body processes
- Haemoglobin- helps transport oxygen, carbon dioxide and nitric oxide
- Enzymes- helps catalyze and control biochemical reactions
- Antibodies- helps immunoglobulins which fend off invading:

  - bacteria,
  - viruses, and other
  - pathogens
  - toxins
  - antigens

Edestin protein is found only in hemp seed. Edestin aids digestion. Edestin protein is considered the backbone of the cell's DNA and is similar to the human body's own globular proteins found in blood plasma. Edestin protein produces antibodies which are vital to maintain a healthy immune system. Since edestin protein closely resembles the globulin in blood plasma, it's compatible with the human digestive system. This may be the reason why there are no reported food allergies to hemp foods. Hemp protein also contains glutamic acid.

Glutamic acid is a neurotransmitter that helps brain function & psychological stress.

Albumin Protein

Albumin is a family of globular proteins. The main protein in your blood is called albumin. All the proteins of the albumin family are water-soluble. Albumin is also a protein made by your liver. Albumin helps keep fluid in your bloodstream so it doesn't leak into other tissues. It also carries various substances throughout your body, including hormones, vitamins and enzymes. Proteins have many important jobs in your body, such as helping to build your bones and muscles, prevent infection and control the amount of fluid in your blood. Albumin is the most abundant circulating protein found in plasma.

Hemp contains 35% Albumin. Albumin protein is another high quality globulin protein and is similar to that found in egg whites. Albumin is highly digestible and is a major source of free radical scavengers. Albumin is the current industry standard for protein evaluation. Digestion transforms hemp protein into amino acids which are the basic building blocks required for the growth and maintenance of body tissue.

Hemp Protein Contains All Of The 20 Known Amino Acids & Repairs DNA

Hemp protein contains all of the 20 known amino acids including 9 essential amino acids (EAAs). These amino acids are labeled essential because the human body can't produce them on its own. A diet that is deficient in EAAs may lead to degenerative conditions.

Hemp Vs Soy & Pea

Hemp is second only to soy in protein content, but when hemp protein is compared to soy protein it should be noted that hemp does not contain trypsin inhibitors that soy does. Trypsin is an enzyme that is essential to nutrition. Since hemp protein is free of the trypsin inhibitor that is found in soy protein, hemp is the king of plant protein. In addition, hemp protein is also hexane-free.

Soy & Pea Hexane Chemical Used In Protein Extraction

Soy & Pea protein is processed with solvent extraction. The solvents commonly used for soy is hexane, which is similar in structure to gasoline. Aside from the use of solvents, soy and pea is not cold pressed for its oil as hemp is. The high heat used to process soy & pea destroys the enzyme functions of the protein. In other words, the protein is essentially "dead." It has lost its electrical charge. Oligosaccharides that are found in Soy and Pea protein. Keep in mind that since soy and pea is a legume and a bean, its oligosaccharide content can lead to unpleasant stomach upset and gas.

Amino Acids

Electrically charged means that the amino acids carry a negative charge. This negative charge is what allows the amino acid to cross the intestinal barrier. So what does this mean? It's what allows your body to uptake nutrients into your bloodstream as the amino acids are the building blocks that are necessary for your body to function. To maintain health, build cell tissue including muscle and to fight off diseases.

Hemp Vs Whey

Whey protein is a popular alternative to soy protein, but it too has disadvantages when compared to hemp protein. Massive consumption of whey protein, by bodybuilders for example, leads to a health condition called intestinal toxemia. The end result is a decrease in muscle gains as it severely damages the ability for the body to maintain an anabolic state. Many bodybuilders who use whey protein experience undesirable weight gain, but it's in the form of a toxic sludge in their gut. This blockage reduces the ability for protein to be absorbed by the body.

Hemp is the highest food source of Edestin protein.

Avocados

Avocados are a fruit that has long been hailed for its anti-aging properties. Avocados are a great source of vitamin E and potassium, as well as monounsaturated fats and antioxidants. The vitamins and minerals in avocados have been shown to reduce cholesterol, improve skin health and lower blood pressure. Avocados are also rich in folates also called folic acid or vitamin B. Folates help with heart attack prevention and reduce the risk of osteoporosis. Avocados also contain oleic acid, a monounsaturated fat that has been shown to lower bad cholesterol, increase good cholesterol and protect against blood clots.

Berries

Blueberries, raspberries, cranberries, strawberries are super rich in antioxidants, such as flavonols and anthocyanins, which promote cell health and can protect against disease. Anthocyanins in particular, found in large quantities in blackberries, are thought to help protect against cancer and diabetes. Darker berries, especially ones that are black or blue in color tend to provide the best anti-aging benefits because they have the highest concentration of antioxidants. According to some studies, blueberries may even help slow or reverse neurological degeneration, improve memory, restrict the growth of cancer cells and reduce inflammation and good for urinary tract health.

Nuts

Nuts are known for the protein they provide, but that's not all these small nutrient-rich foods can do for you. Nuts of all kinds are a good source of unsaturated fats. Like coldwater fish, nuts contain omega-3 fatty acids, which are great for heart health. They're also a good source of vitamins and minerals, including potassium, which helps lower blood pressure; vitamin E, which helps prevent cell damage; and calcium to maintain strong bones. Another great benefit of eating nuts is that they can fill you up without packing on the pounds. That's because up to 20 percent of the calories in nuts doesn't get absorbed by the body, making them a great snack between meals.

Resveratrol

You may have heard that drinking one glass of red wine each day is good for your heart. Well, it's true! The antioxidants and nutrients in red wine can help prevent heart disease by protecting the arteries and the lining of blood vessels. Resveratrol is one of the most well recognized anti-aging components found in red wine and is an antioxidant. Studies have shown that resveratrol may help prevent blood clots, reduce the risk of cancer, decrease inflammation and lower bad cholesterol. White wine doesn't have as much resveratrol as red wine because resveratrol is found primarily in the skins of the grapes. The red coloring in red wine comes from the extra time the wine is in contact with the grape skins, so red wine ends up having more resveratrol than white wine. You can also get resveratrol by eating grapes and drinking grape juice.

Beans Superfood

Beans are good for your heart, the more you eat the more you, well, you get the idea. Beans often get a bad reputation because they can make you gassy, but they're truly one of the great dietary staples. They're an excellent source of low-fat protein, especially for those who don't eat meat. They also contain fiber (which can help lower cholesterol), are rich in antioxidants, and are chock full of all sorts of vitamins and minerals, including iron, vitamin B and potassium. What's more, some beans including soy and kidney beans contain protease inhibitors and genistein, which are thought to help protect against cancer. Studies have shown, for instance, that people who had high levels of genistein had the lowest rates of breast and prostate cancers.

Beans Are A Longevity Super Food

Studies show that white kidney beans which contain carb blockers may be able to aid weight loss. Studies range from 4 to 12 weeks long and the people taking carb blockers lost 2 pounds within 4 weeks and 6 pounds within 12 weeks, on average.

- **White Kidney Beans**

  - White Kidney Beans offer a lifetime of weight control because they contain Amylase inhibitors, also called starch blockers which prevent starches from being absorbed by the body. When amylase is blocked, those carbs pass through the body undigested, so you don't absorb the calories.

Omega's

A popular dietary supplement in recent years has been fish oils, and there's certainly a good reason for that trend. Eating fish, or taking fish oil supplements, provides the body with omega-3 fatty acids that help protect against heart disease, reduce inflammation, decrease the risk of arrhythmia and lower blood pressure. Omega-3 fatty acids are found largely in coldwater fish, including salmon, herring, tuna and sardines.

Studies have even shown that people who eat a lot of fish live longer. One study of middle-aged American men found that those who ate fish two to three times per week had a 40 percent lower mortality rate than those who did not. In men who had previously suffered a heart attack, eating fish twice a week actually lowered their mortality rates by 29 percent

Vegetables

Like fruits, vegetables are one of the best sources of antioxidants available and they can go a long way toward fighting free radicals and slowing the effects of aging. The best vegetables for finding antioxidants are green, leafy vegetables such as spinach and kale. Two of the antioxidants found are lutein and zeaxanthin, which have also been shown to protect against the negative effects of UV exposure. Vegetables are a fantastic source of vitamins and minerals, including vitamins A, C, K and E. They're also great for the immune system, helping the body fortify itself against sickness and disease. Studies have shown that a diet full of vegetables can help prevent cardiovascular disease, lower high blood pressure and, after a heart attack or stroke, lower cholesterol and unclog arteries. Eating lots of veggies (and fruit) could even reduce the risk of cancer in the digestive tract (including the colon and stomach) by up to 25 percent

Grains

Whole grains are good for your digestive system. All that fiber keeps you regular and helps rid the body of unwanted substances, such as bad cholesterol and fats. Fiber also helps control your appetite and keep blood sugar low [source: Beare]. But a diet rich in whole grains, including oats, whole wheat and brown rice, has other anti-aging benefits because they're rich in vitamins and minerals. Eating whole grains has also been linked to a lower risk of heart disease, stroke and diabetes. The key is to make sure the grains you're eating aren't refined, because it's the refining process that strips away many of the essential vitamins and minerals that make the grains so good for you in the first place.

Garlic

Garlic has long been thought of as a healthful and flavorful food, eaten by itself or added into a variety of delicious dishes. Its anti-aging benefits include lowering cholesterol and blood pressure, reducing inflammation, and protecting and maintaining cell health. One of the biggest benefits of eating garlic is that it's a natural way to boost the immune system. Garlic has been used in folk medicine to help prevent and fight against infection for centuries, and scientific studies confirm its benefit as an antiviral and antibacterial food. Additionally, garlic has been linked to helping reduce the growth and spread of cancer cells. Several studies have shown that the more garlic both cooked and uncooked a person eats, the lower their risk of getting stomach or intestinal cancers. It's also been linked to reduced rates of breast and pancreatic cancers. Recent studies of the health benefits of garlic have pointed to hydrogen sulfide as one source of garlic's many health benefits. Hydrogen sulfide is an antioxidant, it relaxes the arteries and promotes blood flow, and studies have even linked it to cancer defense. The body naturally produces hydrogen sulfide, but adding garlic to your diet causes your cells to produce more of this beneficial compound.

Ginkgo Best Circulation And Brain Health Herb

Ginkgo biloba has been used to improve or stabilize mental function, improve memory, and to improve cerebral and peripheral disease. Ginkgo is used for cognitive dysfunction, dementia and Alzheimer's disease. The flavonoid-rich leaves generally improve cerebral blood flow and memory. The ginkgolides inhibit platelet aggregation, while the bilobalide protects against neuronal death caused by global brain ischemia and excitotoxicity-induced damage. The mode of neuroprotection is via antioxidative, anti-amyloidogenic and anti-apoptotic effects. The antioxidative effects of *Ginkgo biloba* are shown by its protective effects against membrane lipid peroxidation. However, vitreous hemorrhage was reported with the use of *Ginkgo biloba* in a patient with age-related macular disease.

Curcumin & Turmeric The Best Anti-Aging Protector

Researchers from the U.S. Germany and India. All agree turmeric is the best supplement you can take as it is virtually an anti-every bad thing that could go wrong in the body. It's anti-inflammatory, anti-carcinogen, anti-tumor anti-bacterial, anti-viral, anti-parasitic and yes, anti-aging.

Losing Fat on an Exercise Program

A nutritional research study suggests that calcium pyruvate can help with weight loss when starting an exercise program. Researchers assigned 23 non-exercising women into two groups: one that took five grams of pyruvate twice a day and the other that took a placebo twice a day. They all exercised for 30 days in a 45-minute walking test at 70% of VO2 pre-training maximum. Results showed the pyruvate group lost almost a pound of fat. The placebo group gained 2.4 pounds of fat.

Aging Facials

Pyruvic acid peels at 50% can potentially become a safe and efficient treatment for facial skin aging, according to a study from *Dermatologic Surgery*. Researchers treated 20 patients with four peeling sessions at four-week intervals. After which, they found skin with smoother textures, less wrinkles and hyperpigmentation lightening. The patients also reported little to no discomfort in the post-peel period.

Hidden Culprits That Accelerate Aging

- **Processed Foods**

  - Fructose- Sweetened Beverages
  - Packaged Snacks (chips, crackers, etc)
  - Preservatives.
  - Packaged Sweets- Candy and sweets are loaded with empty calories, preservatives, additives.
  - Processed Meats- bacon, sausage, cold cuts are loaded with cancer causing nitrates that cause heart disease and high cholesterol.

- **Chemistry**

  - Your body chemistry is composed of acids and alkali in a mineral base, there is a balance to your chemistry that keeps everything in homeostasis. Many substances that we ingest can eventually have an effect on your body chemistry.

Chapter 19

Detoxification Keeping The Fountain Of Youth Flowing

*"Give me the power to create a fever,
and I shall cure any disease."*

Sauna Therapy

Over 2,000 years ago Hippocrates, the father of modern medicine, said "Give me the power to create a fever and I shall cure any disease". Whether this is factual is yet to be determined, although a fever is often the way to trigger the self-healing mechanisms in the body to work to recover from many infectious diseases and additionally help improve the symptoms of age related conditions such as soothing the pain of arthritis, and more. There are a few types of saunas:

- Steam Sauna
- Dry Sauna
- FIR Sauna (Far Infra-Red)

- **Steam Sauna-** Many exotic health and beauty spas of Europe have long revered the steam sauna to provide detoxifying steam and hydrating skin treatments. A steam sauna is beneficial for hydration, aromatherapy, regenerating skin care, detoxification, inducing sweating and the benefits of low grade temperature elevation on the immune system. Steam saunas provide many benefits for health rejuvenation.
- **Dry Sauna-** dry heat creates intense detoxification, within seconds a dry heat sauna can induce sweating and the benefits of low grade temperature elevation on the immune system are phenomenal. Dry heat saunas provide many benefits for health rejuvenation and offer many immunity boosting properties.
- **FIR Sauna (Far Infra-Red)** The sun gives off beneficial rays called Far InfraRed rays, unlike UV rays, FIR rays are very beneficial to human health.

FIR can help rid the body of heavy metal toxicity It also burns stored fat and encourages weight loss.

Health Benefits Of Sweat

A good sweat every day can help rid your body of toxins. Since the beginning of time people have enjoyed the health benefits of natural hot springs and since the discovery of fire, people have been heating water for its therapeutic benefits.

- The North American Indians utilized "Sweat Lodge" as their most effective therapy against disease.
- Ayurvedic Swedenas were utilized by the people of India for centuries and today they still utilize herbalized steam baths as part of the ancient Ayurvedic purification treatment, known as panchakarma.
- In Finland they use sweat therapy in the treatment of chemical dependency due to its purifying effects of perspiration studies show steam treatments can help improve many ailments such as acne and arthritis.

Exercise To Generate Body Heat

Many people exercise just to sweat because exercise is a great way to generate sweat. If you feel worse after exercise it is usually because they are dehydrated or their skin pores and sweat glands may be blocked. If lactic acid soreness occurs after your workout, drink more water and eat magnesium and potassium rich foods to flush out the excess uric acid and it will help increase sweat during your workout.

Heavy Metal Toxicity

Heavy metal compounds are dangerous and they can block the flow of your inner fountain of youth because they are non degradable and last very long in the environment. From the environment, heavy metals enter the human body and cause damage to the brain, liver, central nervous system and other vital areas. Heavy metals weaken the immune system, making it vulnerable to diseases. Heavy metals fuel:

- Cancer,
- Viruses
- Bacteria
- Other pathogenic invaders
- Contribute to the development of diseases.

Toxins Trigger Serious Diseases Such As:

- Cancer
- Alzheimer's disease
- Debilitating chronic diseases
- Fibromyalgia
- Multiple sclerosis
- Adrenal fatigue
- Blood glucose fluctuations
- Hashimoto's disease
- Chronic fatigue
- Chronic inflammation
- Epidemics

The most toxic heavy metals are:

- Mercury (Hg)
- Cadmium (Cd)
- Lead (Pb)
- Copper (Cu)
- Nickel (Ni)
- Cobalt (Co)
- Arsenic (As)

Some heavy metals are necessary for the body, such as copper and cobalt, but only in very small amounts.

Heavy Metal Health Destroyers

While living in this world, it is impossible to avoid everything that is harmful to your health but there are still some things you can do for yourself. Plants help to cleanse your body naturally and pull heavy metals out and help clear the destructive heavy metal residues and reverse the destruction caused by heavy metals, leave a lot of vital nutrients in your body, and rebuild your whole body. There is nothing better you can do for your health by removing heavy metals from your body. One of the best ways to get rid of heavy metals and cleanse your body is to consume all the following seven plants every day while on a monthly detox:

- **Atlantic Red Seaweed** (dulse seaweed, palmaria palmata) Dulse seaweed binds mercury, lead, aluminum, copper, cadmium and nickel. The seaweed also crosses the blood-brain barrier. Unlike other algae, this seaweed is able to remove mercury by itself. It enters the depths and hidden places of the body, finds mercury, binds it and does not release it before leaving the body.

- **Barley Grass Extract Powder** This powerful grass has the ability to draw heavy metals out of your intestinal tract, spleen, pancreas, thyroid, and reproductive system. Barley grass extract powder prepares the mercury for complete absorption by the spirulina.
- **Spirulina** This edible algae draws heavy metals out from your central nervous system, brain and liver, and absorbs heavy metals extracted by barley grass extract powder.
- **Wild Blueberries** Blueberries are small miracle makers as they pull heavy metals out of the brain and cleans places in your body where the heavy metals and toxins are removed. The antioxidants also help repair all your organs This is especially important for brain tissue. It is the most powerful food to help reverse Alzheimer's disease.
- **Dandelion** This plant triggers blood circulation and helps your body to purify from toxic heavy metals, DDT, radiation and other toxins. Dandelion root detoxifies especially organs like the spleen, liver and brain. Dandelion is a prophylactic tool for practically all diseases and is particularly good for the prostate.
- **Burdock Root** Burdock root has the ability to purify toxins from the deepest places of the liver, soften dense and stagnant liver, remove toxic hormones from the liver that have been ingested from external sources such as metals, plastics, herbicides and fungicides. It restores the liver that can be exhausted from Epstein Barr, Herpes Zoster, HHV-6, Cytomegalovirus, harmful bacteria, worms, fungi and other pathogens. The liver is also supported by the presence of phytochemicals in burdock root, which reduce the formation of cysts and adhesions and improve the scar tissue found in the liver, as well as purify the liver lobes.
- **Milk Thistle** Milk Thistle is a powerful plant that supports your liver during purification. It enhances liver resistance, strengthens bile formation and secretion, and has a good effect on the gastrointestinal tract. This plant effectively contributes liver regeneration and promotes liver innervation. Innervation is the supply of nerve impulses to any organ or tissue through nerve cells and nerve fibers, ensuring their connection to the central nervous system. In addition, the milk thistle helps to heal the liver in cases of jaundice and drug or poison damage (including radiation damage).

Cleansing And Detoxification Is A Gradual Process

The purification process depends on how contaminated your body is. To totally cleanse your body from toxins it can take from one month up to a one year.

Heavy Metal Testing & Monitoring

Heavy metals in the body can be measured by a hair sample or lab test via magnetic bioresonance and simple heavy metal tests.

Heavy metals levels could be measured then retested every month, to monitor cleansing and detoxification levels.

Herxheimer Syndrome Side Effects Detox

Some negative side effects of detoxification may occur and it is important to be aware of those side effects prior to beginning your detox plan.

- The most common side effects are:

    o   fatigue,
    o   headaches
    o   diarrhea.

Having high levels of toxins in your body, diarrhea is a normal part of the cleansing process. It will pass. Other side effects may include:

- abdominal pain and gas,
- drowsiness,
- dizziness,
- insomnia,
- nausea,
- vomiting,
- anxiety and
- irritation.

In the case of more severe intoxication, there can be more severe symptom:

- panic attacks
- feeling unwell
- bad taste in the mouth

- rashes

Heavy Metal Toxicity

After exposure, heavy metal toxins eventually spread throughout your body and become toxic. Heavy metals will eventually overload all bodily systems. It slowly affects the excretory system as well as the nervous system. The fact that the body may begin to expel toxins through the skin is also a normal side effect. If the kidney and liver become overloaded with toxins.

To minimize or avoid side effects, it's a good idea to start a detox gradually. This way you will avoid shocking your body too much. Calm, gentle and long-term cleansing of the body prevents the side effects from occurring or these will be significantly less severe. However, if the side effects are too exhausting for you to handle, reduce the dose and wait until the body's elimination has stabilized. Then gradually increase the dose again.

How To Start Body Cleansing Detox

Start with small doses of the detox product, so that your body gets used to the plants.

- Follow the directions on the manufacturer's label, typically, start with 1-2 teaspoons 2 times a day with water or juice for about 1-2 weeks. If you are unfamiliar with algae taste you may add a little juice to your detox drink.
- You can gradually increase your dose up to 4 tablespoons a day. For example, take 2 tablespoons in the morning and 2 in the evening. Because to cleanse your body from heavy metals is a long-term process, there is no need to rush.

Your Diet Plan Can Help Ease Detox Side Effects And Symptoms

Other Detox Recommendations

During your body purification, it is advisable to eat as much fresh and raw food as possible, because it will help to eliminate toxins. For instance, eat foods such as:

- salads,
- fruits,

- vegetables,
- juices, and
- mineral-enriched water.

Drinking Water

It is recommended to drink 1.5 to 2 liters of water per day, which also helps hydrate and prevent headaches. Make warm meals in the evenings. For example soups, stir fries, vegetable cutlets, etc. It is important to be active, to rest and if possible, take a sauna. However, be careful in the sauna, because your body might be weak and there is a risk of fainting. Those who have not done any cleansing before and have not eaten herbal foods at all who have consumed high-fat and processed foods, are advised to begin slowly by gradually reducing the amount of consumed processed foods and coffee. This is to avoid an unpleasant detox crisis.

How To Start Your Day On A Detox

During body cleansing, it is advisable to start the day with warm lemon or lime water (2-3 glasses), to which you can add a grated ginger and a little honey. It helps the liver to excrete toxins produced at night.

- To bind and expel the toxins created at night, you can also drink a glass of fiber water. Follow the directions of the manufacturer's label, basically, add 1 tablespoon of fiber to a full glass of water or juice and drink it every morning.
- In addition to lemon or lime water, it is good to drink raw celery and cilantro/coriander juice every morning.

One head of celery gives you 300-500 ml of raw juice. Celery juice can be made with a juicer. It has the wonderful ability to detox you from a variety of symptoms including chronic illnesses. Celery contains a large amount of useful salts, sodium and potassium, which makes celery juice more alkaline in pH.

Detox Juice

With a daily dose of 500-1000 ml of celery juice, you can quickly restore hydrochloric acid levels. Hydrochloric acids are necessary for the stomach to efficiently break down proteins. If the proteins do not break down properly, it causes putrefaction in the gut, which in turn causes inflammation and diseases. High levels of hydrochloric acid are also important for killing the pathogens that enter thru your mouth.

Water Detoxification Symptoms

However, it is necessary to intake sufficient amounts of water and other fluids. Hydrochloric acid consists largely from water, and if there is not enough water in your body, heartburn will occur because the hydrochloric acid in the stomach is too acidic. Celery juice also increases and strengthens bile production. Strong bile is important for breaking down fats and destroying pathogens.

Celery juice also helps restore the central nervous system, removes old toxins and other poisonous substances such as medicines from the liver and body.

- Drink heavy metal detox smoothie after 30 minutes of drinking celery juice and fresh coriander into the smoothie. It's because coriander enters deep into inaccessible places in your body and extracts the heavy metals of past times. You can always add a handful of coriander to other smoothies, juices or salads.
- Support kidney function with dandelion and field horsetail tea which help lymph work with licorice root tea.

Detox Headaches & Side Effects

Do not start body cleansing if you are:

- Pregnant;
- Breast-feeding
- Hypoglycemic
- Anemic or
- Recovering from an illness

Importance Of Sweating

Each day we are exposed to hundreds of toxic chemicals that are present in the environment. Many pollutants are present in our air, food, soil and water. Environmental pollutants affect us in a variety of detrimental ways:

- Lowered immune system function
- Neurological and neurotoxicity
- Hormonal imbalances
- Organ dysfunction
- Psychological impairment
- Mood disturbances,

- Cancer risk

What Your Skin Really Is

The skin is the largest detoxification organ of the human body. In a healthy person 30% of the body's toxic waste is excreted through the skin. When the skin becomes dehydrated and the pores blocked, the immune system comes under major attack. When this happens waste backs up into the tissues, organs, blood stream, and lymph nodes. Today, because of modern lifestyles, most people show signs of lymph node stress. When the lymph nodes and lymph channels become clogged up. It can be a difficult problem for those suffering from an existing illness and those who are trying to prevent illness. When your skin and lymph system are blocked, your body tissues and fluids become a storage shed for some of the body's most destructive poisons. Toxic blocked cells produce acids that will literally accelerate the process of aging.

Toxins Are The Difference Between Feeling Young or Old / Healthy or Sick

The first step to great health is proper detoxification. The most passive and effective way to accomplish this is through a cleansing detox diet and steam therapy.

Avenues Of Detoxification

Detoxification occurs through the body's natural process of eliminating and neutralizing toxins. Opening the avenues of detoxification is an important step in activating your inner fountain of your via:

- the liver/colon/bowel/feces
- the kidneys/the urine
- the exhalation/the breath and
- the perspiration/the sweat.

"Detoxification Therapy" accelerates these natural bodily processes to help rid the body of chemicals and pollutants and can facilitate a return to a more youthful state of health.

Hyperthermia

Hyperthermia is the raising of body temperature above its normal level of 98.6o F (37oC). It is also known as heat stress detoxification. Hyperthermia is one of the most effective detoxifying treatments available. Most people do not have sufficient energy reserves (oxygen and hydrogen) to create a proper fever to burn off illness, so external methods of raising the body's temperature to facilitate detoxification are required

Detoxification Cleanses Your Inner Fountain Of Youth

Beauty and health are more than skin deep. After a good detox you can truly experience the joy of vital health. You deserve to look and feel great and a good detox plan delivers better health. A daily detox tea can help you have gradual detoxification, also spa therapies that help you sweat, such as using a sauna, will help you internally and detox the skin externally, too.

Benefits of Steam Detoxification

Heat speeds up the chemical processes in the body and induces sweating, making steam bathing one of the simplest and most comfortable ways to rid the body of accumulated toxins. As the pores open up and millions of sweat glands start to excrete sweat, the body rids itself of metabolic and other waste products. Sweat contains almost the same elements as urine, and for this reason, the skin is sometimes called the third kidney. It is estimated that as much as 30% of bodily wastes are eliminated by way of skin through perspiration.

Fat Detox Through Sweat

Induced hyperthermia, through steam, is an effective heat stress detoxification therapy that is one of the only known detoxification programs that is proven successful in removing fat-stored toxins from the body. Heat stress can help remove calcium deposits from the blood vessels and break down scar tissue from their walls.

Heavy Metal Toxins Detox Via Sweat

Studies demonstrate that hyperthermia can remove chemicals such as DDE (a metabolite of DDT), PCBs (polychlorinated biphenyls), and dioxin from fat cells.

However, more than just the common metabolic waste products are eliminated through the sweat process. Natural health practitioners often notice that when heavy smokers get a steam bath or a body wrap for up to 45 minutes their sweat will often leave a yellow residue on the towels. Lastly, steam bathing produces powerful therapeutic effects simply by increasing circulation. The bloodstream plays a crucial role in the maintenance of health as the carrier of nutrients to all parts of the body.

Steam Versus Dry Sauna Benefits

The powerful cleansing and healing process of hyperthermia takes place when the body core temperature reaches between 100 & 101°F with steam and this is accomplished more quickly and more effectively than in a dry heat sauna. It only requires 10 to 15 minutes while relaxing in a steam sauna to reach the goal temperature ranges of 100 degrees. In a 1989 study, researchers concluded that the desired higher heat stress ratings were attained with the use of humid heat rather than dry heat. As the person's temperature begins to rise, the body's natural response is to perspire so that the evaporation of the perspiration will cool the body. Heat loss by evaporation in a dry sauna is considerably greater than in a humid sauna or steam room because in a steam bath, evaporation is not possible and therefore allows little or no loss of valuable body heat. The higher moisture level actually causes condensation on the body to become the primary heat transfer mechanism additionally heating the body.

The effectiveness of steam hyperthermia treatments directly correlates with the ability to eliminate evaporation heat loss during treatments. A steam sauna will cause you to perspire heavily, expelling toxins for a naturally cleaner, healthier you!

Benefits Of Steam Detoxification - A Summary:

- Less time needed to reach and maintain effective temperature levels of 100 Degrees F -101 Degrees F
- The steam effectively washes toxins from the surface of the skin as you sweat, rather than allowing them to dry or bake back onto the skin
- The profuse sweating caused from the steam emulsifies the fat of the sebaceous glands far more effectively than water and clears them of sebum and the bacterial flora they contain
- Keeps the respiratory system hydrated (does not allow for dehydration damage to the delicate tissue of the respiratory system).

Opening The Floodgates To Your Inner Fountain Of Youth

When you detoxify your skin and lymph nodes you open a whole new door your inner fountain of youth and renewed health.

- Environmental Toxins

    Food Additives
    Water Additives
    Personal Care Product
    Chemicals
    Mold
    Pollution
    Smog
    Smoke
    Heavy Metals
    Pesticides
    Herbicides
    Defoliants

While living in this world, it is impossible to avoid everything harmful, but there is still something you can do for yourself. One of the best ways to get rid of heavy metals and cleanse your body is to consume all the following seven plants every day:

Atlantic red seaweed- Dulse seaweed binds mercury, lead, aluminum, copper, cadmium and nickel. The seaweed also crosses the blood-brain barrier. Unlike other algae, this seaweed is able to remove mercury by itself. It enters the depths and hidden places of the body, finds mercury, binds it and does not release it before leaving the body.

Barley Grass Extract Powder- a powerful grass has the ability to draw heavy metals out of your intestinal tract, spleen, pancreas, thyroid, and reproductive system. Barley grass extract powder prepares the mercury for complete absorption by the spirulina.

Spirulina- an edible algae draws heavy metals out from your central nervous system, brain and liver, and absorbs heavy metals extracted by barley grass extract powder.

Dandelion- Is the pretty little yellow flower that grows wild almost everywhere that there is grass, in the U.S. Dandelion is one of god's greatest kidney and liver cleansing plants. Dandelion activates blood circulation and helps your organs to purify from:

- Radiation,
- Toxic heavy metals,
- DDT and
- Many other toxins.

Dandelion root detoxifies organs:

- Kidneys
- Spleen
- Prostate,
- Liver
- Brain.

Dandelion is a prophylactic tool for practically all diseases and is particularly good for the prostate.

Dandelion and Hormonal Imbalances

Dandelion helps cleanse residues, it helps with:

- DHT- a bad testosterone linked to age related hair loss
- Decline in sex hormones
- Stress
- Emotional Mood disorders
- Depression

Natural Hormone Solutions:

- **DIM**
- **DHEA**
- **Adaptogens**

Signs Of Hormone Changes In Women

Many women experience symptoms of hormone loss and struggle with the negative symptoms of hormonal lows and highs. Some of the result of hormonal imbalances are:

- Stress problems,
- depression,

- anxiety,
- severe PMS,
- Mood swings
- Hot flashes
- Night sweats
- menopause symptoms.

But the good news is that natural health supplements, as part of a healthy lifestyle, can help balance your hormones. By the same token, correcting hormone imbalances can make a huge difference in your health, wellness, and quality of life.

How Hormones Affect Your Health

Your endocrine system is a network of hormone-producing glands in your body. It includes your:

- Pineal
- Hypothalamus
- Pituitary,
- Adrenals,
- Kidneys
- Ovaries/Testes
- Pancreas,
- Thymus,
- Heart
- Thyroid.

What Hormones Do For You

Hormones are specialized chemicals that carry messages from the endocrine glands where they're produced to organs and cells throughout your body. Some examples of hormones are:

- Cortisol,
- Adrenaline,
- Estrogen,
- Testosterone,
- Insulin,
- Glucagon,
- T4 and T3

Beneficial Hormone Support Supplements

The most effective supplements for correcting hormonal imbalances in women as well as how to use them to balance your hormones.

- DIM
- DHEA
- Pregnenolone
- Testosterone
- Estrogen
- Melatonin

Hormonal Regulation

Hormones regulate many of your body functions, hormones control your:

- appetite,
- blood sugar,
- energy levels,
- stress response,
- sleep schedule,
- sex drive,
- sexual function, and
- fertility.

Hormone Imbalance Signs

The following list of signs and symptoms that indicate a hormone imbalances for women:

- Sleep issues
- Fatigue or tiredness
- Reliance on caffeine to get through the day
- Poor memory or concentration
- Mood problems (irritability, depression, or anxiety)
- Appetite changes
- Weight gain or loss
- Sugar or carbohydrate cravings
- Becoming "hangry"
- Temperature sensitivity
- Facial hair

- Low or erratic sex drive
- Bloating or water retention
- Enlarged or tender breasts
- Aches and pains
- Irregular menstrual cycles
- Heavy or prolonged bleeding
- Hot flashes
- Vaginal dryness
- Infertility
- Headaches
- High blood pressure
- Rapid heart rate

If more than a couple of these items ring a bell, you may have problems resulting from a hormone imbalance. However, you can fix your hormone levels and reduce the symptoms of hormone imbalances. You don't have to live with tiredness, mood issues, or low libido.

Every hormone imbalance is slightly different–therefore, you should experiment with lifestyle changes, including health supplements, to see what works best for your situation.

Bottom Line About Hormones

Your hormones affect your overall health in significant ways. Stress, mood, libido, PMS, and the severity of menopausal symptoms can all be influenced by your hormone levels. Your endocrine system is complex, but you can use natural supplements and other lifestyle changes to improve your hormonal health. However, if you are suffering from severe hormone imbalance symptoms, you should speak to an endocrinologist or other trusted healthcare practitioner.

The benefits of balancing your hormones include:

- Slow aging
- Enhanced youthful vitality
- Reduced cravings,
- Better blood sugar levels,
- Greater energy,
- Less stress, and
- improved fertility.

- Increased Longevity

An aging body has changed in many ways, and not just in those obvious to visual inspection. The typical old body is identifiably different from the typical middle-aged body at the level of cells, genes and biochemistry: biochemical processes, gene expression, levels of molecular damage, cellular behaviors, cellular populations, and so on.

High Cholesterol & Atherosclerosis

Damage to mitochondria leads to oxidation of low-density lipoproteins (LDL), which in turn leads to detrimental changes involved in atherosclerosis, which is the principal cause of coronary heart disease and other forms of cardiovascular disease. Most modes of biochemical wear and tear contribute to a wide range of recognized age-related conditions and frailty.

The Goal of Activating Your Inner Fountain Of Youth Is To Slow The Causes of Aging.

Age Related Cell Loss & Targeted Gene Therapy

Some tissues lose cells with advancing age, like the heart and areas of the brain. Stem cell research and regenerative medicine provides very promising treatment options for degeneration through cell loss. Scientists are perfecting how to eliminate the telomere-related mechanisms that lead to cancer by selectively modifying telomere elongation genes by tissue type using targeted gene therapies.

DNA Repair

Mitochondrial DNA is outside the cellular nucleus and accumulates damage with age that impairs its critical functions. Gene therapy to help mitochondrial DNA copy properly into the cellular nucleus. Other strategies for manipulating and repairing damaged mitochondrial DNA are developing every day.

Systemic Enzymes

Some of the proteins outside our cells, such as those vital to artery walls and skin elasticity, are created early in our life and recycle very slowly. These long-lived proteins are susceptible to chemical reactions that degrade their effectiveness. Scientists have discovered systemic enzymes or compounds to break down problem proteins that the body cannot handle.

Brain Health Amyloid Plaque

As we age, junk material known as amyloid accumulates outside cells. Immune therapies are currently under development for Alzheimer's, a condition featuring prominent amyloid plaques, and similar efforts could be applied to other classes of extracellular junk material. Tripeptidyl peptidase 1 (TPP1), cuts these junk plaque precursors formed by peptide fragments called amyloid-beta into pieces. The findings suggest that increasing TPP1 activity is an innovative target for treating Alzheimer's disease. TPP1 can effectively break down peptides associated with Alzheimer's disease that are normally very resistant to degradation.

How To Get Rid Of The Junk

Junk material builds up within non-dividing, long-life span cells, impairing functions and causing damage. The biochemistry of this junk is fairly well understood; the problem lies in developing a therapy to break down the unwanted material required. One source that is a potentially safe and suitable non-toxic option is microbial enzymes found in soil bacteria, this is one example that could produce effective results that could be safely introduced into human cells.

Cellular Senescence

Cellular senescence is a permanent growth arrest caused by telomere dysfunction, the critically shortened telomeres that arise after many cell divisions and failed DNA replication errors and also by other kinds of stress such as genotoxic damage.

Bio-gerontology Cellular Senescence

One of the active controversies in the sub-field of bio-gerontology is the treatment of cellular senescence and while senescence certainly arises as cells get older in culture, we are still figuring out how senescent cells contribute to age related decline in tissue function, it's not fully clear, yet, as how to make the body prevent senescence or to what extent the phenomenon actually plays in physiological aging.

Nanotechnology Cellular Senescence

The buildup of senescent cells accounts for a significant fraction of tissues in later life, the engineers should already be looking at nanotechnology approaches to eliminate the accumulation of senescent cells in this day and age of targeted therapies for discriminating cell destruction and other advanced biotechnology under development.

Chapter 20

Your Inner Fountain Of Youth Plan In A NutShell

You can best activate your inner fountain of youth by following a healthier lifestyle. Your lifestyle must include healthy habits and how healthy your habits are is a key factor in how long you will live and will greatly determine the quality of life and longevity you will have throughout the course of your lifetime.

"Alcohol Accelerates Aging"

Much of the research points to oxidative damage as the main cause of aging. DNA copying errors are a very creative force in the aging process, these errors are highly destructive for the individual as it causes declining health and disease. Therefore, you must take measures to repair DNA damage and to help reverse the aging process. The following help prevent DNA damage and are the keys to activating your inner fountain of youth.

- **Quit Bad Habits**
  The single best thing you can do for your health and longevity is quit all your bad lifestyle habits before they kill you. If alcohol is a problem, be sure to read my other book, "Quit or Die The truth About Alcohol". The following are some other bad habits you should consider quitting if you plan on living a long and healthy life.

- **Health Care**- Get regular healthcare checkups and follow a healthy preventive medicine plan. Find a doctor who specializes in geriatrics or anti-aging. your new doctor may recommend yearly assessments and testing of various biomarkers, including lipids, DHEA, estrogen, cortisol, thyroid, lung function, and micronutrient level monitoring.

- **Beauty Sleep**- Get your beauty rest. Sleep is not just for beauty. Your body needs down time to repair cells as the body only repairs itself during the deepest state of sleep. Your mind needs dreaming to process life's experiences each night to stay sane.
- **Quit Smoking**- If you smoke quit smoking. Smoking has been indicted for a laundry list of ills from heart disease to lung disorders, all of which can foil your longevity plans.
- **Quit Drinking**- Drink only in moderation. Alcohol infiltrates every cell of the drinker's body, damaging genes, wrecking havoc and inflaming your liver. The old adage that a glass of wine a day for women and maybe two for men, is false. Read Quit or Die to find out why.
- **Lower Bad Fat Intake**- cut down your saturated fat intake,
- Increase Good Fat Intake- eat avocado, wild caught salmon fresh coconut to increase heart-healthy omega-3 fat intake.
- **Lower Red Meat Intake:** eat less red meat and when you do choose a lean-cut. Avoid commercial beef unless it is non-gmo grass fed and all organic.
- **Avoid Sweets**- choose whole fruit with almond milk whip cream instead of cake and ice cream;
- **Carb Up**- consume more complex carbs, such as whole grains, fruits, and vegetables instead of chips, cookies and crackers.
- **Increase Fish**- The healthy fats in wild salmon, mackerel, and sardines help keep oxygen free-radical molecules from damaging your cells.
- **Portion Control**- watch your portion size and eat in moderation. Your stomach is the size of your fist, so only eat that amount to limit risk of overeating. your total food intake calories should be around 1500 for weight loss 2000 calories to maintain current weight and 2000+ calories to gain weight.
- **Fasting For Longevity**- Studies in rats show that a 30% calorie restriction means longer life.
- **Lose Excess Weight**- rhesus monkey studies show life extension in years from a reduction in food the conclusion is losing excess pounds means maintaining a healthy weight results in a longer healthier lifespan.
- **Precursor Hormone Replacement**- the natural steroid, DHEA is a precursor hormone to many other hormones including testosterone. DHEA is often recommended for aging. However, there is less evidence that DHEA has rapid anti-aging benefits in comparison to HGH.
- **Sex Hormone Replacement**- The replacement of sex hormones such as, testosterone, estrogen and progesterone can be beneficial but keeping the levels in a safe range can be complicated. There has been massive research studies on sex hormones. The replacement of these hormones must be

monitored closely to stay in safe level ranges as the combo therapy may increase, rather than cut, the risk of cancer and heart disease.

- **Growth Hormone Replacement Therapy-** Be careful when tweaking your hormones such as HGG. "There have been big studies to determine the relationship between decreases in human growth hormone and symptoms of aging and growth hormones have been shown to combat against:

  o thinner bones,
  o body fat,
  o mood swings
  o muscle loss

Giving growth hormone can have negative side effects, too. HGH has been shown to cause:

- water retention,
- carpal tunnel syndrome,
- high blood pressure, and
- blood-sugar fluctuations.

Anti-Aging Steps To The Fountain Of Youth

Supplement- Most of us suffer from overconsumption and malnutrition at the same time. Too much of the wrong things, and not enough of the right things. Many people take a fistful of vitamins and minerals, every day. The American Medical Association endorses taking a daily multivitamin. In addition to the effective antioxidant vitamin C, Co-Q10, vitamin E, alpha lipoic acid

Attitude- stay positive about growing into a ripe old age, with a youthful mind set. A study at Yale recently showed that those with a positive view of growing older lived seven years longer than those who resisted it.

Mind Set- Guilt and regrets are part of the past and drag your energy, mind and happiness down. Evolving and changing is how we stay young. Keep a young mindset.

1. Don't be afraid to make a big change.
2. It's never too late to move,
3. Try an adventure, join the Peace Corps or a club
4. If you're bored, change careers.

5. Have a happy relationship, but don't keep bad company
6. If you're not happy, don't be afraid to make a change
7. Never say you're too old,
8. Bad decisions need to be changed.
9. Plastic surgery can be life-enhancing but as a last resort
10. Do what it takes to look and feel better,
11. Change your life overnight.
12. Never retire. Its debilitating
13. Take some time off for a vacation
14. Do something useful.

Prevention Of Age Related Diseases

Aging, a characteristic systemic modification of biomolecules, causes the increased susceptibility of an organism to develop disease. Among various diseases, arthritis is one of the most prevalent diseases of the elderly.

Age Related Diseases

The mechanism by which aging of biomolecules perpetuates adult onset illnesses involves a variety of risk factors. Numerous studies indicate that oxidative stress, characterized by free radicals, mediates biomolecular deterioration, depolymerization of glycosaminoglycans, somatic mutation involving DNA oxidation, lipid peroxidation and protein cross-linking. Depletion of antioxidant reserves is involved in a wide array of pathophysiologic conditions and thus plays a crucial role in the etiopathogenesis of common age related diseases such as:

- Arthritis- the exact mechanism behind its involvement in such events is not yet fully understood and needs further investigation. Furthermore, in the past few decades, it has been emphasized that exogenous supplementation of antioxidants delays the age-mediated destruction of the joints.
- Cardiovascular disease- is a general term used to encompass any disease of the heart and/or blood vessels. These diseases range from stroke to atherosclerosis and heart failure. Age is a major risk factor for cardiovascular disease, along with smoking, diabetes and poor diet. All of these factors have a common feature: they increase the levels of oxidative stress. Much is known regarding oxidative stress, aging and the development of cardiovascular disease, but the precise pathogenesis and mechanisms of this trifold relationship remains complex.

- Diabetes Prevention- the epidemic of diabetes and cardiovascular complications has also soared simultaneously, particularly in the elderly population. Type 2 diabetes is a predominant factor for aging and is closely associated with the degeneration of different organs in the human body. Breakdown of cellular homeostasis, and oxidative stress, play a significant role in the development of type 2 diabetes, and they also contribute to the aging process. Impairment of glucose metabolism as a result of type 2 diabetes also generates reactive oxygen species (ROS) in cells and tissues; ROS eventually damage cellular organelles and accelerate aging in diabetic patients. Type 2 diabetes may not be the sole factor for aging but it promotes the process in association with other macrovascular and microvascular complications such as retinopathy, neuropathy, nephropathy, cardiovascular diseases and cognitive impairment. Healthy living in older age requires systematic prevention of diabetes and better management of oxidative stress-induced and associated complications known as 'metabolic syndrome'.

Spiritual Health

When discussing human health we must recognise well being goes well beyond the mind and body. A person needs spiritual food, too. Spiritual nourishment is important no matter what your religion.

The God Gene & Believers Lifestyle

The God gene is a hypothetical hypothesis that proposes human spirituality is heredity influenced by a specific gene, scientists have named "vesicular monoamine transporter 2" (VMAT2). Researchers believe the VMAT2 gene predisposes us humans to being spiritual or more capable of mystic experiences.

People who work on their spirituality and find joy in faith strengthen their god gene. There is peace in the word of god that no other thing can give a human. Faith and prayer are scientifically proven to work. Multitudes of people have experienced healing of serious diseases throughout the world by the power of prayer. The bible says, God is the great almighty healer, those that believe it lives healthier longer lives.

A God Loving Spirit & Spiritual Lifestyle Ensures A Longer, Happier, Healthier Life

When you live by the word of god there are no regrets. There is a sense of less stress when we turn all life's problems and worries over to God. For some believers, they feel their longevity is totally in God's hands; for others it is attributed by living a godly lifestyle, therefore, longevity is not achieved by faith alone, it is a combination of their faith, lifestyle and diet. For example, The long living Seventh-Day Adventist of Loma Linda, California tendl to live well beyond their eighties, 10 years longer than the average American lifespan and they attribute their living a long life by being obedient in their diet. They even have a profit-like diet coach who mentors them on good diet habits and many of them are mostly vegetarians. However, some Adventists choose to eat certain "clean" meats, such as fish, poultry, and red meats other than pork, as well as other animal products like eggs and low-fat dairy. Other Seventh-Day Adventest around the world do not eat pork, rabbit, or shellfish as they are considered "unclean" and thus are banned in the Adventists diet. We can learn alot from the Adventist.

Religion & Diet

Some religions require periods of fasting and prayer. Many religions have strict diet rules for example, Hindi peoples worship the cow and most would never eat cow meat and their products are sacred. Hindus see the cow as a particularly sacred and generous, docile creature, one that gives more to human beings than she takes from them. The cow, they say, produces five things: milk, cheese, butter (or ghee), urine and dung all which they use for the healing of their culture or for cultivating. Hindus who do eat meat eat other meats and not beef. The respect for cows is part of Hindu belief, and most Hindus avoid meat sourced from cows as cows are treated as a motherly giving animal, considered as another member of the family.

"Kosher" describes food that complies with traditional Jewish law. Orthodox Jewish peoples eat kosher foods and especially on Fridays, on Shabat kosher meat and fish. Certain foods, notably pork and shellfish, are forbidden; meat and dairy may not be combined and meat must be ritually slaughtered and salted to remove all traces of blood. Observant Jews will eat only meat or poultry that is certified kosher.

Millions of Catholics around the world eat fish on Fridays as part of a religious observance. Orthodox Christians, who follow the Julian calendar, and observe Lent, are more strict, as the faithful are expected to abstain from meat, meat by-products, poultry, eggs, and dairy products for the entire lent period.

The list of other religion's food restrictions goes on and on and it is something to be respected when dining with or serving multicultural friends and guests.

Moses And The Nile

The Pharaoh's daughter in the story of the finding of Moses is that she found him in "the giver of life" the Nile. She named him Moses, saying, "I drew him out of the water." Later in life Moses had other miraculous encounters with water. Moses stretched out his hand over the sea, and the Lord drove the sea back by a strong east wind all night and made the sea dry land, and the waters were parted. Later, Moses was told, by God, to take the rod he had used to part the waters of the Red Sea and strike the rock at Horeb, from which water would come out so "that the people may drink" (Exodus 17:6). God has a supernatural power over water and our inner fountain of youth.

God Made Our Body's To Be Comprised Of 70% Water And More Than 70% Of Earth Is Covered In Water, Also

Biblically The Longest Living Humans Documented:

1. Moses- 120 years old
2. Methuselah- 969 years old
3. Adam- 930 years old
4. Enoch- 365 years
5. Abraham- 175 years old
6. Isaac- 180 years old

The bible tells many clues of how these long livers lived and they were all men of faith. God commanded his people to fast one day a year, on the Day of Atonement in Leviticus 16:29-31 God commanded the observance of the Day of Atonement. There are many benefits of short water fast. It has taken scientists until now to figure out how to stimulate Autophagy for the body to self-clean.

God Commands Us To Fast For Good Reason Now We Know Why

The Water And The Everlasting Fountain Of Youth

When we do short fast we still drink water. The body needs adequate water and can only survive a few days without water. Water is another name for life. Drinking it is not limited to the usefulness of water. The bible reference has another meaning. The "Water of Life" in Revelation 21:6 as spoken in the word of the prophets of God say: "And he said unto me, It is done. I am Alpha and Omega, the beginning and the end. In the English version bible, it says: "To all who are thirsty I will give freely from the springs of the water of life." In KJV it says: "I will give unto him that thirst of the fountain of the water of life freely."

"We are all spirits here, having a human experience"

Will Humans Ever Become Immortal

The idea of becoming immortal has always been a fascination to humans since the early fountain of youth, explorers. We know that we can follow the new anti-aging methods and live a longer life in a more youthful state of health. As of yet, scientists have not cracked the immortality code. However, bible believers have always believed there is an opportunity to become immortal and enjoy eternal life. In the bible, John 3:16 of the new testament, the bible says: "For God so loved the world, that he gave his only begotten Son, that whosoever believeth in him shall not perish, but have eternal life". According to the bible Jesus is the eternal fountain of youth, Jesus is the water of life, he is the everlasting fountain of youth. Currently, immortality is achieved by living a godly life and taking daily soul-saving measures according to your faith. In the bible, heaven or hell are places of eternal life. Each place is described very differently and how you live is a personal choice that will determine where you will end up in eternity. Basically heaven is described as a happy place with God and hell is a punishment of eternal separation from God. There is no way to explain it all in this book but if you haven't read the new testament I encourage everyone to read it and make their own choice and to learn more about eternal life beyond this one.

Pure Live Water Is A Key Solution To Activate Your Inner Fountain Of Youth

In the meanwhile, during this lifetime you can enjoy a longer life by following a healthy anti-aging lifestyle. As of now, no human is immortal but, someday there may be health discoveries that allow us to live as long as methusalem and beyond, more secrets are yet to be discovered but as research continues we discover more ways to activate your inner fountain of youth. To be continued...

References:

Wikipedia
Harvard Medical School Research Archives
NIH- National Institutes For Health
CDC- Centers For Disease Control
UCLA- Health Research Archives
John Hopkins- Health Research Archives
Cornell University Health Research Archives
New England Journal of Medicine
The Holy King James Bible

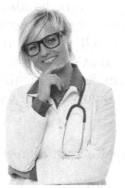

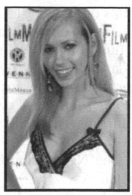

Dr. Joy St. Peters, PhD

Summer Perry, CHT,
Geriatrics Research Contributor

Author Biography:

Joyce Peters, PhD- is a pioneer in Anti-Aging since its inception. Dr. Joy helps many famous celebrity clients maintain their stunning appearance and youthful vitality by utilizing the tips and techniques as revealed within. Dr. Joy completed postgraduate studies at some of the nations top universities, including Harvard Medical school and has worked in some of the most prestigious plastic surgery and wellness clinics coast-to-coast. Dr. Joy is the author of numerous self-help books. You can learn the secrets that help her Hollywood clients look years younger than their actual age. Now, you can do these fun treatments at home, and look and feel years younger and achieve a better mind and body, too.

Summer Perry- Is a medical student, researcher and contributor. Summer works at UCLA medical center and has worked with some of the finest medical professionals in the field of genetics as well as collaborating with the anti-aging product manufacturing companies. Summer is a co-formulator of several anti-aging products. She is a member of the Phi Theta Kappa socicty and carned her BS in health sciences. Summer continues her studies in Genetics, Geriatrics, Anti-Aging and Preventive Medicine.

About The Book: Hidden within your own body, is an internal fountain of youth. Learn what many celebrities pay thousands for to help them look years younger than their age and how you can activate your own inner fountain of youth, too. Discover how to activate your own inner fountain of youth and enjoy a safe, effective, healthy lifestyle and self-care beauty system that really works. Discover how to reset your

Age-Clock with tips on how to slow aging and turn back the hands of time to activate your inner mechanisms of youthful vitality. Scientists have discovered these simple daily rituals to flush out old cells, stimulate new cell growth, regenerating home beauty therapies and newly discovered substances that slow down and help reverse the signs of aging. You can prevent the cause of wrinkles and repair DNA damage for a healthier and longer life. The key to unlock your own youthful vitality, beauty and longevity is at your fingertips.

- Discover The New Compounds That Help Reverse Signs of Aging & Slow Your Age-Clock
- Anti-Aging Secrets For Looking & Feeling 10+ Years Younger Than Your Actual Age.
- New Beauty Treatments You Can Do At Home To Tighten, Tone & Lift Aging Skin.
- How To Eliminate Hidden Culprits That Cause Wrinkles and Accelerate Aging.
- How To Repair Your DNA And Lengthen Your Telomeres
- How To Prevent The Cause Of Wrinkles & Do An At Home Face-Lift
- The Keys To Living A Longer, Healthier And Happier Life.
  Bonus:
  Your Genes & The 7 Sirtuin Factors To Prevent Disease
  Your Epigenetics & NutriGenetic Correctors
  Your Blood Type And The Right Anti-Aging Diet
  Your Body, How To Strengthen & Regenerate It

Printed in the United States
By Bookmasters